JONATHAN CHAMBERLAIN was brought up in Ireland and Hong Kong, where he lived for many years working as a teacher and writer. His previous works include *Cancer: The Complete Recovery Guide*, and his website on cancer-related issues is *www.fightingcancer.com*. He has also written *Chinese Gods, An Introduction to Chinese Folk Religion* and *King Hui, the man who owned all the opium in Hong Kong*. Jonathan is also the founder of two charities: The Hong Kong Down Syndrome Association and Mental Handicap Network China Ltd.

CANCER RECOVERY GUIDE

15 ALTERNATIVE AND COMPLEMENTARY STRATEGIES FOR RESTORING HEALTH

Jonathan Chamberlain

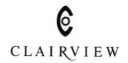

CLAIRVIEW

For Bernadette

Clairview Books
Hillside House, The Square
Forest Row, East Sussex
RH18 5ES

www.clairviewbooks.com

Published by Clairview 2008. Reprinted 2008

A catalogue record for this book is available from the British Library

ISBN 978 1905570 14 0

Cover by Andrew Morgan Design
Typeset by DP Photosetting, Neath, West Glamorgan
Printed and bound by Cromwell Press Limited, Trowbridge, Wiltshire

Contents

Disclaimer

The information contained in this book is not intended to serve as a replacement for professional medical advice. Any use of the information is at the reader's discretion. The author and publisher specifically disclaim any and all liability arising directly or indirectly from the use or application of any information contained in this book. A health care professional should be consulted regarding your specific situation.

Acknowledgements

This book is the result of a long journey that started when I borrowed my first book from the resource centre set up by the Hong Kong Cancer Fund. To them I am forever indebted. I must also thank the hundreds of authors and researchers whose work I have benefited from. The battle for truth in the world of cancer is ongoing. The power of the pharmaceutical companies must not be underestimated. Everyone who has contributed information to any alternative health internet forum has helped to resist this power. This book has benefited from many of these contributions of knowledge and experience.

On a more personal level, I would like to acknowledge the help and support of Margit Whitton and Louise Aylward who have kept me on track; Leonard Rosenbaum for his promptings and suggestions; Jack Gontier who forced me to restructure the information I had and in doing so opened up the possibility for this book to be written; Dr Shamim Daya who introduced me to a number of new therapies; and Sevak Gulbekian for agreeing to publish this book, recognizing that it is an important contribution to the national debate on orthodox versus alternative therapies in the case of cancer.

Preface

You have been diagnosed with cancer, or someone close to you has been; or you are wise enough to prepare for that possibility well in advance – because who knows when it will strike? You, along with everyone else in North America and western Europe, currently have a 40–50% likelihood of getting cancer at some time in your life and it makes sense to know what your options are.

For me cancer can be likened to a juggernaut hurtling down a narrow road. If you keep your eye on it you have some chance of not being hit.

My reason for writing this book is to give you a quick run-through of the major strategies that are being followed in the area known as complementary or alternative medicine (CAM); in the case of cancer, I believe these strategies to be far superior to the orthodox strategies (surgery, radiation and chemotherapy). This is not because I am opposed to western medicine, which is far superior to any alternative when it comes to dealing with physical trauma, for example. But it has not proven to be very successful against cancer. The reason for this will become clear as the discussion progresses. The fact that there are so many alternative approaches out there is a clear demonstration that there is a big problem with the orthodox approach. If doctors could cure cancer there would be no need for this over-abundance of alternative approaches. And as this book will make clear, many of these approaches make very good sense. Indeed you will read in the following pages a number of stories of people who used alternative methods to cure their cancers.

Many people equate, in a dismissive way, alternative medicine with, in the words of a friend of mine, 'New Age nonsense'. By this they mean that it is wishful thinking, that it has the savour of anti-scientific mysticism. This assumption needs to be quashed right from the start. All of the approaches described here in this book are based on solid science or observation or credible experience.

Before I begin, I'd like to introduce myself and explain how it is I came to write this book.

Thirteen years ago my wife Bernadette was diagnosed with cancer. She did what we all thought was the sensible thing. She followed the advice of the oncologists. She underwent exploratory surgery followed by radiation and chemotherapy. She was dead a year later. She could not have died quicker if we'd done nothing. And that year was a year of great pain for her as she suffered through her treatments – and great pain for me as I sought desperately and fruitlessly to find some route to a cure in the books I found in the bookshop, the library and the local cancer support centre.

Eventually, I came to realize that the book I was looking for didn't exist. I wanted a book that would take me by the hand and tell me what all the options were, what their rationales were and why there were problems with the orthodox approaches. So I wrote *Fighting Cancer: A Survival Guide.*

Since then, far more information has become available – the internet has exploded – and over the last two years I have spent a great deal of time updating the book. The result is now so comprehensive that I feel no hesitation in retitling it *Cancer: The Complete Recovery Guide.* (For details see *www.fightingcancer.com.*) But at more than 500 pages this may seem too burdensome a read – especially for those of you who are desperate for a quick answer to the question: What should I do now?

Cancer Recovery Guide is the book for you now. *The Complete Recovery Guide* can wait until you are more settled and comfortable with your changed circumstances.

I am absolutely convinced that Bernadette would be alive today if, firstly, I knew then as much as I do now and, secondly, I could persuade her of that fact.

That last sentence encapsulates the central quandary that many cancer patients – along with their families and their friends – are faced with. The person doing the research isn't necessarily the person who needs to make the decision.

On the one hand, there is the problem of knowing what to do (there are many options); on the other, there is the problem of how to get this information to the person who needs to make the decision. In the end the decision has to be made by the person who has the cancer and everyone else needs eventually to accept that fact – but they would be deficient in their love and friendship if they did not seek to influence that decision.

One thing that I have learnt over the years responding to readers of my book and visitors to my website is that we are all different. We approach problems in very different ways. Our upbringing, environment and our own individual character will all have an enormous impact on our decision-making. Therefore, for me to say to you, 'do this or do that' is very likely to be counter-productive. One person will be attracted to machines that zap, another will want something natural, fragrant – the essence of a plant or flower, perhaps. One person will want facts that have been proven 'scientifically' before choosing a therapy; another will be happy to do something on the basis of a risk-cost-benefit analysis, irrespective of the formal validation. If the risk is low, the cost is low and the potential benefit high, then many people – myself included – will be happy to go along with a strategy even if there is no definite proof that it will work. In any case very few strategies will work 100 per cent all of the time. Very few have been sufficiently researched for any proof or otherwise to be ascertained. That's just a fact that needs to be factored in.

Also, there is the fact that not one of us is biochemically 'normal', i.e. sharing characteristics with 95 per cent of the population. This is a statistical certainty. That is, we all have biochemical aspects that place us at extremes, that are rare. What works for 95 per cent of the population may not work for us. To put it simply, we are all biochemically unique.

When it comes to making decisions, some people are confident in their ability to choose a course of action, while others are so lacking in confidence that they are permanently uncomfortable and want an expert to make the decision for them.

One truth, however, unites us all. Whatever decision we eventually make is our own responsibility – even if we choose to pass this responsibility on to an expert. The buck stops with us. It therefore makes sense to educate ourselves, and all education must start somewhere. I have written this book to give you a quick orientation of the strategies underlying various complementary and alternative approaches to cancer. My hope is that once you have read this book you will begin to breathe easier. You will relax. The fear and the panic will recede. My message to you in a nutshell is this: there is hope, real, solid-as-granite hope. Some people have found their cancers disappearing 'miraculously'. Cancer treatments don't need to be painful or devastating to your health. You can get well again – and you can do so painlessly, though it may take a little willpower.

Now let us look at what this book can achieve. *Cancer Recovery Guide* tells you what 15 strategies you can put into practice right now. You don't have to begin all of them. Indeed some conflict with others. Nevertheless, these 15 strategies will help you think about how you want to proceed. You will be in charge over what it is you want to happen. This in turn will help you get over the immediate panic of cancer, so that you can take the time to read other books which will give you a more in-depth understanding of cancer and the options available.

Finally, I do need to make a statement. The law requires it. The object of this book is to provide information – not to be a substitute for professional care. Because each person and each situation is unique, none of the approaches and treatments mentioned in this book is advocated for any specific individual.

My best wishes go with you.

Jonathan Chamberlain
Brighton, England
November 2007

Introduction:

Understanding the Basics

Before we go on to the 15 Strategies we need to establish what cancer is, what the word 'cure' really means and what the pros and cons of the orthodox therapies are: the surgery, radiation and chemotherapy that, almost certainly, you have been, are being or will be pressured to undergo.

What is cancer?

Most people have a vague understanding of what cancer is, but the closer they are to the reality of it the more they find their understanding to be inadequate. It is very important to understand what cancer is. So what is it?

If you ask an oncologist for an overview of cancer he is likely to say something like the following. Cancer is an umbrella term for a large number of diseases – anything up to 2000 or more. Each of these separate diseases has its own unique biology and needs to be attacked (treated) in its own distinct way. However, the common feature of all these diseases is that, at their heart, they manifest the uncontrollable growth of malignant cells. A cell is malignant if it has lost the ability to die through natural programmed cell death (a process known as apoptosis) and spreads easily to other parts of the body, so spreading the disease. This is the characteristic that distinguishes malignant from benign tumours.

Viewed in this way, we can see that the malignant cells are seen as an enemy. They are simply something that needs to be eliminated. An analogy is that they are foreign invaders — like the Martians in H.G. Wells' book *War of the Worlds*. The best way to deal with them is to kill them, blast them, excise them, poison them, and nuke them. And that is what the orthodox methods of cancer treatment essentially seek to do.

This is not the only way to look at cancer, however. Holistic therapists conceptualize cancer in a different way. They say the malignant cells are not the disease. They point out that cancer cells are not foreign invaders. Rather, they were originally the body's own normal stem cells that have — for some reason — not progressed normally to become normal tissue cells but have instead progressed abnormally and become cancer cells. Something has happened to the cells to make this happen.

Up to this point, everyone is in complete agreement. But the orthodox oncologist will say the problem lies within the cell, in the very heart of its DNA. It is, in short, a cell with genes which for some unknown reason that we shouldn't bother our heads over have become evil and deviant — a problem of a mutation that has given birth to a malevolent child — and therefore the cell needs to be eliminated.

Hold on, says the holistic therapist. Not so fast. You've skipped over the key question. Cells don't become cancerous for no reason and we don't buy the explanation of a random, sudden, inexplicable mutation. If mutation is the trigger, then some outside factor has pulled the trigger. It is the body itself, the metabolism of the surrounding cell tissues that causes the cell to change. Put simply, a cell growing in a healthy environment will continue to grow in a healthy way. A cell growing in an unhealthy environment is going to become deviant. It becomes deviant precisely because this is the only way it can survive in the context of the surrounding unhealthy tissue. So, if we change the environment from a state of ill health to a state of good health, the cancer cell can also be returned to a normal cell again.

Simply returning the body's tissues to a healthy state can cure cancer, according to the holistic therapist. From this we can see that the holistic therapist views the cancer cells as symptoms of a disease, not the disease itself. If that's the case, what is the disease? The disease is simply this: the unhealthy state of the body. The nature of what 'unhealthy' means in this context will be examined later.

Another way of putting this is to say that cancer is not an evil and alien enemy. It is in fact a friend, a friend in disguise perhaps, but nevertheless a friend. A friend that is signalling furiously that there is a big problem.

The idea that cancer is a friend may surprise you. But for those who see it — and see it truly — not with foreboding but as a wake-up call, this is a natural response. The actor Mandy Patinkin has written: 'The greatest thing in my life was getting cancer because it taught me how much I love my life, my family, my friends and my work. And it taught me that I must find some peace and calm every day. I never could sit still long enough to meditate, but [now] I do it every day. I'm like a little baby Zen Buddhist.'

Does it make sense to shoot the messenger? Does it make sense to ignore the message?

This conflict of views over the root causes of cancer – mutation versus metabolism – has powerful implications for us. We need to know what the problem is before we can usefully go in search of a solution. If we are to cure cancer we need to know what we are expecting that cure to do.

From the oncologist's point of view the only matter of any importance is to kill the malignant cells. But from the holistic therapist's point of view this is really nothing but a confidence trick. Let's say the oncologist succeeds in killing all the cancer cells – what then? The underlying cause has not been addressed. The unhealthy metabolism will give birth to new cancer cells, which will then have to be zapped again. How many times is the patient going to be able to handle this amount of punishment (and these treatments *are* punishing)? In fact, most of those looking for alternative cures are people who have already been through the orthodox system. Second time round they know they don't want to go through it again.

The holistic therapist takes the view that the malignant

cancer cells will heal themselves in some way, generally by reverting back to normal cells and then immediately triggering their own death (apoptosis), but only if we can return the body itself to a state of health.

The way I like to visualize this conflict is in that children's story of how Summer and Winter argued over who was stronger. They decided to see which of them could make a man take his coat off. Winter went first and blew cold winds and freezing rain at the man, but this only made the man clutch his coat tighter. No matter what Winter did, it couldn't persuade the man to take his coat off. Then it was Summer's turn and instead of attacking the man it simply shone brightly and made the whole world warm. Now the man gladly took his coat off. Winter tried to succeed by attacking the man; Summer succeeded by changing the environment.

What does 'curing cancer' really mean?

Now that we have looked at the different ways of viewing cancer, let's consider what it means to 'cure' cancer.

The traditional view of a cancer cure is that you go to the doctor and undergo the treatments he or she provides. Then you keep your fingers crossed and hope it works. You return to your old way of life – your diet and your habits, your work schedule and your relationships – in the hope that you will be able to preserve these unchanged.

But if you go with the holistic therapist it is precisely your old way of life that needs to be changed – and changed forever. Your diet will need to be overhauled. Your exercise regime may need to be enhanced. Your emotional life, even, may need to be re-examined. Why? Because it is precisely this old way of life that has resulted in the whole body becoming toxic, and so stimulating some of the cells that are most vulnerable to this toxicity to change and become malignant.

For many people this is too complicated or exhausting to contemplate. They would rather maintain their old way of life at all costs. To a large extent people feel defined by their habits and attitudes. They would rather just go along with what their doctor tells them to do. And doctors often tell their patients to carry on their lives as they always have. 'Should I change my diet?' At most, they may suggest that adding some fruit and vegetables would be beneficial. Wise patients soon come to realize that doctors are so closed to any suggestion that diets or supplements can be curative that they stop discussing it with them. The result is a widening chasm. Since 1990, in the USA, more money has been spent on alternative therapies than on mainstream medicine – a subject that is causing great disquiet to the editors of the medical journals that have reported this trend. Yet most patients do not feel they can discuss what they are actually doing with their doctors.

People feel vulnerable. Many patients convince themselves that what the doctors are doing is backed by science. In fact this is not true. It is well known – and well accepted even among the medical profession – that 80% of what doctors do has no scientific backing. That is the figure that is regularly mentioned in medical journals. Many common surgical and medical procedures have simply not been compared with the benefits of taking a placebo in a double blind clinical trial, which, in the world of medicine, is the scientific gold standard. In addition, much of the science that supposedly supports many drug related treatments is 'massaged' – to put it politely – in such a way that it cannot be relied on. And many drugs are used in ways that have no evidential backing. These are well-known flaws that doctors know about but patients remain ignorant of.

Many people who have cancer don't simply want to be passive recipients of their doctors' expertise. They want to do something, they want to feel in some way in control, that they can affect their own fate and not simply be a victim of it.

These are enormously important issues and each person will need to think through their own position very carefully. For myself, if I ever get cancer I will know that it is my own lifestyle that is to blame. I will know that I have to change my lifestyle, permanently. If I don't change it, the cancer will return. Of this I am certain. To put it as bluntly as I can, if you think you can simply get rid of the tumour and then go back to your 'normal' way of life then you are living in a fool's paradise. The cancer is a sign that the way you have been living is unhealthy, in one or more key respects. If you can identify the problems and rectify them then you are more likely to live to the age of 100.

Understanding the pros and cons of standard treatments

Since it is clear that I am in favour of alternative therapies, I should explain briefly what I see as the main problems associated with orthodox therapies. First of all, it must be clear to anyone who has followed the news that, despite great advances that seem to be announced every other week, there are in fact no new wonder cures. Quite simply, orthodox medicine doesn't, for the time being at least, have the answers. People are continuing to undergo surgery, radiation and chemotherapy in very large numbers, and months or years later many are dying from the disease.

So, what are the pros and cons of surgery, radiation and chemotherapy?

Surgery

Pros:
If the surgeon can cut out all the tumour and a margin of healthy tissue and there has been no spread of cancer cells to other parts of the body, then simple surgical excision will amount to a cure (until the circumstances that gave rise to this tumour give rise to another one). Benign tumours can be

safely removed. Sometimes surgery is necessary – such as in the case of brain tumours – where the limited space available means a growing tumour, even if benign, will inevitably cause brain damage. Occasionally surgery to reduce the size of a tumour, known as debulking, is considered to be useful.

Cons:

Firstly, any cutting into a tumour, either for diagnostic purposes (a biopsy) or during surgical removal, is almost certain to release cancer cells into the blood supply where they are taken to other parts of the body. Surgery may therefore directly lead to the spread of the cancer.

Secondly, any cancer tumour large enough to be visible is already in an advanced state. It is very likely already to have spread cancer cells to other sites. When this happens the main tumour appears to exercise some control over the growth of the other tumours. When the main tumour is removed this control also ceases. It is often the case, therefore, that a few months after 'successful' surgery on one tumour, a number of other tumours suddenly appear in other places.

A third problem is the possibility – in many cases the virtual certainty – of long-term health impacts as a result of surgery. In the particular case of surgery to remove a colon cancer, a significant section of the colon is likely to be removed. This will mean a lifetime of digestive problems, almost certainly severe enough to interfere with any future attempt to maintain good health through dietary means.

Since diet is the foundation of good health and of central importance in all sensible alternative anti-cancer approaches, this consequence is devastating – although rarely factored in to the decision-making process.

Another problem with surgery is that it takes place in hospitals and these are becoming very much more dangerous places to be, especially for people with cancer who can be assumed to have compromised immune systems. The risk of infection from one of the dozens of viruses and bacteria that are now endemic in surgical units – MRSA and all the others – is very great. These infections can kill.

How to protect yourself:

If you do elect to have surgery then you need to protect yourself as far as possible. One way would be to take increasingly large doses of vitamin C, up to 20 or 30 grams (20–30 × 1000 mg) a day. Don't worry, no amount of vitamin C will cause toxicity. If the body takes in too much for its immediate needs it dumps the rest by causing a sudden bowel movement – the amount needed to cause this response is known as the bowel tolerance level. The sicker you are the higher this will be – a good sign that the body needs vitamin C to fight illness. However, you should build up your intake slowly by one or two grams a day, and maintain the desired level throughout your stay in hospital and for some time after. I deal later in this book with the question of what form of vitamin C is best (see page 99). At this point let me just say that the bright orange effervescent tablets that dissolve in water and taste of fizzy orange are possibly the worst possible way – just think of the sugar and artificial flavourings and colourings! Lavender essential oil is also a great healer and anti-microbe agent. It can be lavishly rubbed into the body on and around scars without having to be diluted. Magnesium supplements are also extremely helpful for healing and tissue repair. Magnesium citrate (1000 mg per day in divided doses) is recommended.

Radiation

Pros:
Ionizing radiation is a powerful killer of anything in its path, given the right conditions.

Cons:
The first problem with ionizing radiation is that it is only 100% effective against cancer cells if surrounding healthy cells are also killed. Damage to surrounding organs is therefore inevitable. This can have very serious consequences, in the pelvic area especially. The consequences can be so serious as to make life barely worth living. I detail some of these stories in *Cancer: The Complete Recovery Guide*. Some people are living with such damage from radiation that their lives have been effectively destroyed. Sometimes these consequences do not appear for many years.

Secondly, areas that have been irradiated cannot subsequently be operated on as the body's ability to heal is severely compromised.

Thirdly, radiation is more effective in areas of high oxygenation, but cancer cells typically occur in areas of low oxygenation. There is therefore a great likelihood that radiation will not kill all cancer cells at which it is directed.

Fourthly, cancer tumours that have survived exposure to radiation are very likely to become both more aggressive and more resistant to control by other means. This means the cancer spreads faster than previously and is much harder – though not impossible – to stop.

The effects of radiation damage may not be immediately obvious. Heart attack rates among breast cancer patients irradiated on the left side are far higher than for women who were not so irradiated. Haemorrhaging caused by the rupture of blood vessels weakened by radiation can also occur 10 or 20 years after the event. Lastly, radiation when used against brain cancers causes a slowing down of mental processes, amounting in some cases to mental retardation.

How to protect yourself:
Supplementation with potassium and iodine or, alternatively, taking large doses of seaweed products is very beneficial. Another suggestion is to take large doses of vitamin C and 800 iu of vitamin E (alpha-tocopherol succinate, not standard vitamin E) to reduce local swelling. Transfer factors, extracted from colostrum, have also helped relieve the side effects of

radiation and chemotherapy. The hormone melatonin and the herb St John's wort taken at night can also help recovery. Aloe vera gel should be rubbed on irradiated skin.

Iodine, usually in the form of potassium iodide, is getting a lot of new attention as a cancer treatment and preventative – especially in relation to breast cancer (but it is almost certainly of value for all cancers). No one really knows why iodine is useful – though it has long been used as a way of purifying water. Perhaps it is an anti-fungal, perhaps it interferes with cell replication, and perhaps it boosts the thyroid gland in an important way. Most people tested are found to be iodine deficient. The suggested doses are 2–4 × 12.5 mg tablets per day for three months, then gradually reducing the dose to 1 × 12.5 mg tablet a day when normal health has been resumed. (For more information and for a cheap source, go to *www.breastcancerchoices.org*.) You should know that current medical textbooks take the view that such doses are toxic. Refer your doctor to the articles on this website for a clarification of the reappraisal that is currently in progress.

Dr Albert Szent-György, the Nobel Prize winning biochemist who isolated vitamin C, wrote: 'When I was a medical student, iodine in the form of KI (potassium iodide) was the universal medicine. Nobody knew what it did, but it did something and did something good.' In those days the standard dose was 1 gram, which contains 770 mg of iodine.

Chemotherapy

Pros:

Some cancers have shown a very positive response to chemotherapy. It has been very effective in the treatment of the following cancers: Burkitt's lymphoma, Hodgkin's disease, non-Hodgkin's lymphoma, acute lymphocytic leukaemia, choriocarcinoma, embryonal testicular cancer, Ewing's sarcoma, lymphosarcoma, retinoblastoma, rhabdomyosarcoma and Wilms' tumour. Unfortunately, together, these account for only 5% of all cancer cases. Even in this short list, chemotherapy is variable in its effectiveness. For testicular cancer doctors are now claiming a higher than 90% cure rate, but for adult leukaemia effectiveness is less than 50%.

Cons:

For all other cancers, including all the major cancers, the benefits of chemotherapy are considered to be marginal — a few percentage points at best. Given the extent to which these figures are massaged in the first place, this is effectively saying that chemotherapy has little or no impact. Despite much hyped wonder drugs like Herceptin, chemotherapy is not effective against breast cancer in any meaningful sense. One example of how the benefits of drugs can be hyped is to say that people taking this drug have a 33% higher chance of being cured compared with other drugs. If other drugs claim to have a cure rate of 2% (which is more than most do!) then this means that the absolute benefit rises to 2.7%, less than

1% improvement in real terms. (This is the situation with Herceptin.) The sad fact is that out of 100 cancer patients, around 75 will be given chemotherapy but only 3 will in fact benefit.

Chemotherapy, like radiation, also makes cancer tumours more aggressive. The standard scenario is that the doctors give chemotherapy (even when it is not particularly useful), the cancer tumour shrinks for a while, and the patient thinks the cancer is in remission. But then the tumour starts to grow again – and much more quickly. Despite further chemotherapy sessions this growth is unstoppable. The patient dies.

Chemotherapy is extremely damaging to your health. No chemotherapy agent has been developed that will only attack cancer cells while leaving normal cells alone. If it has been designed to attack fast growing cells then it will also attack the cells that lubricate all our internal tubes. This can cause major problems for our urinary system to take one example.

Most chemotherapy regimes are more painful than you can possibly imagine.

How to protect yourself:
Some chemotherapy drugs are toxic to the heart. Very large doses of coenzyme Q10 (300–400 mg a day) should be taken to help protect the heart. Vitamin C in large doses may also be helpful. Although many oncologists insist vitamin C will interfere with the effectiveness of the chemotherapy, this has not been supported by research.

A special note on brain cancers

Brain cancers pose a very specific problem for two reasons. The first is that the brain is in a very confined space and any treatment that causes swelling or inflammation will result in the brain pressing against the bone casing of the cranium and this will cause brain damage. This problem applies equally to the alternative treatments. Great care must be taken to choose therapies that do not cause inflammation. The second problem is that there is a blood-brain barrier that prevents many chemicals from going up to the brain.

In the case of brain cancers, whether because of the cancer itself or the treatment, there is almost certainly going to be what doctors carefully call 'neurological deficits', i.e. damage to mental functioning. This may simply reflect itself in a subtle slowing down that is barely perceptible or it may lead to more serious mental retardation. It should be noted that children who undergo chemotherapy for any cancer will be similarly affected.

Summary

Most patients are naturally dependent on their doctors for treatments that are 'scientific'. The problem is that any impartial assessment of the facts strongly leads to the conclusion that most orthodox treatments for cancer, while they may (or, more likely, may not) be 'scientific', simply don't work and are at the same time highly damaging to the patient.

For myself, if I ever get cancer – though I hope I am doing enough to keep it at bay – I have already made the decision that I will only consider these orthodox options once all other avenues have proved unsuccessful. Even then, I cannot imagine that I will be persuaded. Perhaps it is better to live with a slow growing cancer than to attempt treatment that is very likely to make it more aggressive. There is statistical support for this position. One researcher, Dr Hardin Jones, Professor of Medical Physics at the University of California, came to the conclusion in the 1960s that you were on balance likely to live four times longer if you did nothing for your cancer than if you did something. This conclusion has never been decisively challenged in the four or five decades since then.

*   *   *

Let us now turn to the 15 strategies that I believe can help you recover from your cancer – without any damaging side effects. These do not need to be taken in a consecutive order. Indeed, you may choose to ignore even a majority of the strategies. They are simply options. Each one is a potential journey. Only you know which of these strategies makes sense for you personally.

And you almost certainly have time to read this book and consider your options thoughtfully. Don't let the doctors panic you into making a decision. Unless you have one of the very rare, highly aggressive cancers, you certainly have time – let's say one or two months – to think through the consequences of your decision and to try out some of the alternatives. In fact, you could be cancer free within six weeks from now. I can't promise you will be. But some people have become cancer free within six weeks of following an alternative therapy.

You have time to consider the options because your cancer has been growing a long time already. It has been growing for years. The older you are the longer you have, because the older you are the slower the cancer is growing.

This brings me to one last point that needs to be repeated. The information in this book is not to be taken as medical advice. You, and you alone, must assume responsibility for your own decisions.

Many people feel frightened by this burden of responsibility. Fear is often the result of ignorance. The future is dark. Every decision appears to be threatening. 'What happens if I am wrong?' you might ask yourself. We can never be sure that things will work out well. When we choose to marry someone we cannot know that it will not end in divorce. All we can do is justify our decision by saying: 'This is what makes most sense to me now.' And that is all we can say when it comes to choosing a treatment for our own cancer.

But for things to make sense there must be some clarity. In reading this book, you will, I hope, become clearer as to why you have cancer and what you can personally do to get rid of it. And of course any decision can be changed at any time. And deciding for orthodox treatments doesn't necessarily mean you have to decide against the alternatives.

The 15 Strategies

The 15 strategies in the following pages are options intended to enhance your understanding both of the complexity of cancer and of the variety of strategies that alternative methods seek to employ. I have ordered them as follows:

Strategies 1–4: focus on mental, emotional and, in a loose sense, spiritual approaches to healing.
Strategies 5–9: focus on the body with a view to returning it to a state of health.
Strategies 10–14: focus on the cancer itself and ways of eliminating it.
Strategy 15: focuses on support and sources of further information and help.

While Strategies 1–5 can all be immediately activated in parallel, some care needs to be taken not to practise too many of Strategies 6–14 simultaneously. Many of the suggested approaches are potentially curative on their own. If you do too many at once the cancer can break down too fast and overload the system, poisoning it. Some people have died from this toxic crash on what is usually a very weakened system. Go slowly. Once a cancer has gone into reverse, i.e. started to shrink or die off rather than grow, then victory becomes inevitable if we can maintain that direction. If you do wish to combine therapies then phase them in slowly so that there is an incremental increase from week to week rather than doing everything maximum strength all at once. In short, please be sensible and patient.

Strategy 1:

Embrace Hope — Cancer is Curable

When my wife Bernadette learned that despite all the surgery, radiation and chemotherapy her tumour had returned (it went from invisible to five inches long in a matter of months), she was informed that she had three months to live. She was told this on 17 January. She died on 16 April. Three months exactly. Was this just a good prediction on the doctor's part or had Bernadette died on schedule because her trust in the doctors was so great that when they gave her three months to live she, consciously or unconsciously, took them at their word?

The first lesson we need to learn from this is that we need to be very careful of the messages we receive. Negative messages — if allowed headroom — can be very dangerous to our long-term health, happiness and well-being. We call this the power of 'nocebo'. Nocebo is the negative form of the more commonly understood term 'placebo'. It acts like a voodoo curse. For many people the word cancer is so entwined with the idea of death that the consequences seem inevitable. My job in this book is to tell you very firmly that this needn't be the case. Cancer is a wake-up call, for sure. But that's all it is.

The problem with assuming the worst is that it can be self-fulfilling. If there's no cure for cancer, some people tell themselves, why bother to do anything? If there are cures, the doctors will tell us about them. If the doctors don't sanction a course of treatment, then that course of treatment must be unscientific and therefore worthless. This is the argument that many people use to comfort themselves to the grave. I find it very sad. Let's look at this argument point by point.

1. If there's no cure, why bother to do anything?

Let me say this emphatically: there are cures. Dozens of cures. In this book you will read about Pattie who used a particular herbal compound on her breast cancer – and the cancer tumours bled out of her body over the next month. She is alive and cancer free today. Anne Frahm had only weeks to live when all treatments had failed to rid her of her terminal-stage cancer – she had even undergone a bone marrow transplant. She changed her diet and only five weeks later she was free of all signs of cancer. She went on to live another ten years. Her story is told in the book *Cancer Battle Plan*. Then there is Beata Bishop who in the early 1980s was found to have malignant melanoma, one of the fastest progressing and most intractable cancers known to man. She is alive today, 25 years later, and is cancer free – all because she persevered with a diet that doctors to this day dismiss out of hand. These are real people. Beata Bishop wrote her story in her book *My Triumph Over Cancer*. Michael Gearin-Tosh's book *Living Proof* tells the story of how he was diagnosed with a type of cancer that is generally considered incurable, how he refused all orthodox treatments and how he cured his cancer with a combination of diet and vitamin C therapy – he was to die eleven years later but, and this is very important, he did not die of cancer!

I want to emphasize one point very clearly: Anne Frahm, Beata Bishop and Michael Gearin-Tosh were all diagnosed as terminal cancer cases before they turned to alternative approaches. They cured themselves of *terminal* cancer, that is to say cancer that has spread widely throughout the body and which was, in each case, considered incurable by orthodox means. If they can do it, you can.

2. If there are cures why haven't they been tested?

Cancer research is extremely expensive. Pharmaceutical companies directly or indirectly fund most research. It's obvious that pharmaceutical companies have no interest in proving that some natural product or a diet can cure cancer. There are no profits to be made from any product that is not patented – not the kind of profits that pharmaceutical companies want. They owe it to their shareholders to make profits by selling drugs. Indeed, like every other public corporation they are obliged to maximize profits and to oppose anything that will impact on those profits. (Read Joel Bakan's book *The Corporation* if you are in any doubt about this matter.) They are not particularly interested in cures; they are, however, very interested in profits. They are certainly not interested in unpatentable natural substances; they are only interested in patentable drugs.

This is possibly the best definition of the difference between the orthodox sector, on the one hand, and the alternatives, on the other – one depends on patented drugs while the other is based on unpatentable substances or therapies.

Turning to the 'independent' cancer research charities, we should ask why they are not funding research into areas that are not patentable. They certainly should be. The fact that they aren't is a scandal.

3. If there are cures why aren't doctors telling people about them?

There are a number of reasons. Firstly, doctors are heavily influenced by the pharmaceutical companies. In fact a slew of books written by ex-editors of various medical journals have recently appeared criticizing the medical profession for the degree to which it has let itself be co-opted by the pharmaceutical industry: Jerome Kassirer's *On The Take, How medicine's complicity with big business can endanger your health* (Oxford University Press, 2005); Marcia Angell's, *The Truth About the Drug Companies, How they deceive us and what to do about it* (Random House, 2004), etc. The titles of these books make the point with absolute clarity. These books are published by major, highly reputable publishing houses.

Secondly, mainstream doctors have little or no formal training in diet. One doctor told me that the last time he had read anything about vitamin C was in high school – it hadn't appeared on any of his medical courses.

Thirdly, doctors in some countries – this applies particularly to the USA – can be struck off the medical register and their licence to practise can be taken away if they recommend diets or supplements to cancer patients. In some states, the treatments of surgery, radiation and chemotherapy – ineffective and dangerous though they are – are mandated by law, as 15-year-old Abraham Cherrix, from Chincoteague Virginia, discovered in 2006. He had already had chemotherapy for his Hodgkin's disease but when he discovered it wasn't working he decided he wanted to quit and investigate the alternative approaches. The Department of Social Services decided that as a juvenile he did not have the right to make that decision, and that if his parents aided him then they were guilty of negligence. Fortunately, six months of litigation ended with a negotiated compromise. But other children in the USA have been kidnapped from their homes and forced to undergo unwanted and damaging treatments.

So, to summarize the situation so far: there are cures but doctors can't tell you about them (because they don't know about them) or they won't tell you (because it would endanger their professional position to do so).

This is a situation that reduces many otherwise sane people to paroxysms of purple fury. It is outrageous. But let's not get too focused on the negatives. Let's look at the positives. The personal stories quoted in this book establish beyond doubt that there are cures. There are ways of eliminating cancer and making sure it doesn't come back – and this can be achieved without damaging the body.

We've already looked at 'nocebos'. Let's turn now to the positive power of placebo.

When pharmaceutical drugs are tested for efficacy, they are compared with inert pills called placebos. This is to see if the drug has a measurably greater effect than the placebo. What is interesting about these tests is that the placebos themselves have a positive effect. How is that possible? A pill containing nothing of any recognized medicinal value can have a positive impact on a medical problem – and this is not a weak effect. It can be measured at anything from 20–50% of a placebo group experiencing the benefit. The key point is that they don't know they are taking a placebo. There is a possibility that they are taking the drug. It is the psychological power of hope, of possibility, that has created the beneficial results.

Hope itself is potentially curative. Interestingly, this placebo effect does not appear to be connected to any consciously held positivity on the part of the person taking the placebo. You don't have to mutter to yourself: 'I will get better. I will get better.' Indeed, that can be counter-productive as I will explain in a later chapter.

Here's a story of a placebo cure. A three-year-old boy with a severe case of whooping cough was seen by the doctor. The doctor appeared before the boy in great robes. He sat on the boy's bed and peeled a peach – no doubt chosen because it was an exotic fruit. Then he sugared it and cut it into small pieces. He fed each piece slowly to the boy. As he did so he told the boy that he was going to be fine, that the peaches would make him well again. He made the boy feel that health was inevitable. However, on leaving the room he told the father that he did not hold out much hope for the boy. The whooping cough was so serious it was almost certain to be fatal. The next day the boy was still alive and the doctor came again. As before he made sure he was wearing his impressive medical robes. As before, he fed the boy personally with some fruit. After 40 days and 40 visits the boy was well again. The boy's own subconscious mind had harnessed the resources of his body to cure himself of a disease that was considered to be almost certainly fatal. Whatever the processes involved, this is very powerful medicine.

The doctor in this case was the famous Sir William Osler and the boy was the brother of Dr Patrick Mallam, who published the story in the *Journal of the American Medical Association* (December 22, 1969). Osler, incidentally, is famous for his comment: 'In today's system of medicine a patient has to recover twice: once from the disease and once from the treatment.'

I will end this section with a story that Deepak Chopra tells. A woman came to him with severe stomach pains. She was operated on and found to have rampant cancer. There was nothing they could do for her. However, not wishing to upset her, Chopra didn't tell her about the cancer. He told her they had found the cause of the problem and removed it. Many years later, he was surprised to be visited by the same woman. She laughingly told him that the previous time she had been sure she'd had cancer and was so embarrassed at finding it was something minor that she had told herself sternly not to be silly, to forget about it and just get on with life. When Chopra did tests he found that she was indeed cancer-free. In her case, the belief that she didn't have cancer was enough to cure the cancer.

Felicity Corbin-Wheeler

Felicity Corbin Wheeler is a Reader in the Church of England who has an international biblical-based Health Ministry with its centre in Portugal. Having lost a daughter to cancer, despite what she refers to as 'the "best" of orthodox medicine', she began to research the importance of nutrition in cancer. She eventually came to the conclusion that the answer to nutritional therapy is firmly based on 'what God tells us to eat in Genesis 1:29–30'. In September 2003 she herself was diagnosed with terminal pancreatic cancer. Of all cancers this has one of the worst prognoses. Death usually follows quickly. However, she did not give up hope, but put her faith in 'the living enzymes in the seeds that God tells us to eat when He creates us, and the seed of the apricot has natural cancer cure qualities of hydrocyanic acid. This is also known as amygdalin, or laetrile, which has been given vitamin status as B17 because the seeds are vital for health.'

She not only ate the seeds but, in order to get the maximum dose of laetrile, she undertook a series of 13 intravenous laetrile treatments given by a doctor sympathetic to her approach – two other doctors had refused to do so – followed by a daily intake of B17 tablets (she obtained her supplies of laetrile from www.cytopharma.com). The dose levels had been worked out for her at the Oasis of Hope clinic in Tijuana, Mexico. Believing God's Word about the importance of the seeds, and having complete faith in the course she was following, she expected to be healed. 'I was in constant prayer and I was prayed for by many people.' Within four months scans showed the tumour shrinking, and within a year there was only a scar left. Felicity has told her story in her book *God's Healing Word* and she has a website at www.felicitycorbinwheeler.org

Harness the Healing Power of the Mind

Cancer is almost certainly the direct result of a way of living and being that is unhealthy in some key respects. We need, therefore, to change our mentality and our attitudes if we are to overcome the disease. The power of placebo discussed in the previous chapter demonstrates very clearly the enormous healing power that the mind can have. How we can harness this power is the subject of this chapter.

As we shall see in more detail when considering Strategy 6, a state of low tissue oxygenation is held to be the key cause of cancer. It is easy, but a mistake, to see this as simply a fact relating to the physical body. The truth is a state of low oxygenation has an impact on the whole person. Herbalist Ingrid Naiman describes the following impacts on a person suffering from low oxygenation:

The symptoms of poor oxygenation include pallor and fatigue, poor circulation to the extremities (cold hands and feet), and sometimes dizziness or mental fuzziness. The psychological symptoms are subtle: lack of fortitude, an easy sense of defeat, conviction that the effort needed to do

something cannot be made, vulnerability, and perhaps even some disorientation.
(*www.cancerchecklist.com*)

The truth is mind and body are one. The body affects the mind and the mind affects the body. We can conclude from this that all thoughts are as much facts as physical symptoms. If our mind and body are one then our body is intelligent and our thoughts are physical. Or we can say that the mind is a reflection of the body, and the body a reflection of the mind. This leads me to the following conclusion: if the body is diseased in some way, then we cannot say that we have the disease but rather that the disease is part of us, part of our identity. We are the disease and our behaviour is an expression of the disease.

This at least is the position of the famous health guru, Deepak Chopra. The point of contact between the mind and body are the neuro-peptide transmitters – the body's 'messenger molecules' as Chopra calls them. Contact between the mind and body is via the neuro-peptide transmitters – the body's messenger molecules. These spring into existence at the touch of a thought or emotion. But where they come from no one knows. All that is known is that non-matter is transformed into matter.

Chopra calls the zone where this occurs the '? zone'. This question mark zone is a place below the visible. It is a world where quantum rules dictate reality – and one of the rules is that things can happen suddenly, absolutely and inexplicably, the so-called quantum leap where A can become B instantaneously.

The most important technique for harnessing the power of the mind is meditation. There are a number of different types of meditation, but here I will focus simply on the form of meditation that involves focusing the mind on the breath. The idea is to sit in a quiet place, in a comfortable, relaxed but erect posture, and let the mind follow the out-flow and the in-flow of the breath. Paying primary attention to the out-flow has been shown to have the impact of increasing the volume of the in-flow of breath, and since we wish to improve the oxygenation of our tissues this is an important physiological effect. However, meditation has many other benefits. Psychologically, it is calming and has been shown to improve contentment. This psychological benefit is the result of the change in the brain-wave patterns that occurs during deep meditation. And since stress is such an enemy, any way of aiding relaxation is to be welcomed. Half an hour of meditation in the morning and, if possible, again in the evening will be time very well spent.

Another form of meditation involves visualization. Visualization is a technique of calling to mind a scenario and simply staying with that image for as long as you can and as often as you can. For example, you may decide to see the cancer as an enemy. You visualize the cancer as a balloon and then you imagine the balloon to be under attack from a thousand darts which pierce the skin so that it slowly deflates and eventually disappears. If this image is too aggressive for you, you may wish to see the cancer as a flower that gradually withers and dies, or a friend that you put on a train and say goodbye to. Only you can say what kind of image seems most fitting for you. But whatever the image, replay the same visual narrative ten or more times a day. Close your eyes and talk to the tumour. Tell it to go away and leave you in peace.

If you don't feel you can summon up an intense enough image you might draft out the kind of narrative you want to hear, and go to a hypnotist. Ask the hypnotist to put you into a hypnotic state and to read the narrative. Or tell the unconscious mind what is expected of it, to help you to get better and to help the cancer go away.

Self-hypnotism is a useful halfway house between these two options. There are books on the subject, or you can ask a hypnotist to teach you techniques.

In a hypnotic state you normally remain perfectly conscious and aware of what is going on. As Richard Feynman, the Nobel Prize winning physicist, once commented, it feels like you can open your eyes at any time and come out of the state. It's just that you don't feel like doing so. It is not the blank, trancelike state that is so often depicted in films.

I started this chapter by noting the impact of the body on the mind. Ingrid Naiman explained why ill people often find it difficult to persevere. This is an important point. The herbalist Dr Richard Schulze has a 30-day diet that he claims is curative for many conditions, including cancer (see his book *There Are No Incurable Diseases*). However, he believes that at most 10% of those who start on it actually finish. As someone who has given up smoking the hard way – going cold turkey – I can comment from experience. I knew I wanted to give up because I knew that my habit – 40 unfiltered cigarettes a day – was going to kill me before I got to the age of 60. This thought so obsessed me that I saw that even if the tobacco itself wasn't going to kill me the voodoo power of 'nocebo' very likely would. I just had to give up. This was in the days before the Carr programme or nicotine patches. Time after time I would get to three or four days without a cigarette only to capitulate. It was on the fifth time in twelve months of trying that I eventually succeeded. And one of the tricks I used was to just take each day at a time. I would say to myself: I can keep doing it today; I won't think about tomorrow. In fact, the idea of giving up completely was such a problem that I promised myself that I would have another cigarette when I was 60 and reconsider the situation. Somehow that took the panic away, and once I'd hit three weeks I knew I'd succeeded.

Sometimes we have to trick the mind. By tricking the mind we trick the body. We need to give ourselves small, immediate goals that we can achieve and not scare ourselves with the big goal. Keep telling yourself: I can do this for another day, another meal, another hour.

Ian Gawler

In 1975, Ian Gawler, a 24-year old Australian veterinarian, was diagnosed with bone cancer. He underwent surgery and had his right leg amputated. He was told that he had only a 5% chance of surviving for five years and that if the tumours returned he would only have a few months. The cancer did return later that year.

Deciding to take a pro-active approach, Ian and his wife went to the Philippines, where Ian received treatment from several folk healers. On his return to Australia, he decided to follow a diet, take up meditation and explore a wide range of natural therapies. He believed the secret lay in stimulating the immune system and to let go of stress and anxiety.

He won his battle and the cancer went away. To this day he remains healthy and cancer free. He wrote a book, *You Can Conquer Cancer*, and set up the Gawler Foundation, based in Melbourne, to provide cancer support programmes for anyone seeking to follow the alternative path.

He attributes his success to the fact that he took responsibility for his condition and recognized that he had been responsible for causing it. By taking responsibility he felt in control and believed that he had the power to reverse it.

In an interview with the journalist Beryl Rule he said: 'Psychologically, the big need is to change. If we recognize that a particular pattern has aided in creating the disease, then obviously a new pattern is required... The disease creates the excuse for change. It produces a new situation or insight that allows the patient the space to change their rigid patterns.'

For more information go to *www.gawler.org*.

Love and Forgive Yourself and Others

Cancer is, alongside everything else, a journey of the emotions. It is very easy to look at the physical manifestations of cancer and to treat them simply on the physical plane – whether mechanical or biochemical. But if we look at the emotional aspects of cancer simply as side notes there is a danger we will miss something important.

Many of us carry around anger – often anger that we cannot express and so we turn it inwards on ourselves. Or there is despair. Life may seem meaningless and empty. We may feel locked into a relationship or job that we don't want, or locked out of paths to the future or ways of living in the present that we feel are of vital importance. For psychotherapist Lawrence LeShan, these toxic emotions can be the seed-bed of cancer.

In traditional Chinese medicine (TCM) the body is seen as having channels of energy – meridians – that connect head and feet and various organs and systems in between. In a healthy situation the energy flows freely. In an unhealthy situation there are blockages at various points. While there does not appear to be any obvious physical entity that corresponds to these channels and no outer proof of their existence, nevertheless we do know that acupuncture works in ways that are inexplicable without this theory.

The idea that the body is a system of flowing energy is important for the point I wish to make in this chapter. Emotions that are blocked will have a negative impact on the body's energetic system, and this in turn will have an impact on the health of organs or systems in other parts of the body.

We all know the sense of release we get when some pent-up emotion is allowed to be released. The relief when we discover we have passed an exam, the flow of happiness when a dispute is amicably settled, the sense of empowerment we get when we choose a course of action that is important to us.

I have a very strong memory of the moment I first saw my first child, my daughter Stevie, who I had already been told almost certainly had Down's syndrome. You can imagine how dismayed and unnerved I was at this news. The gush of pure love that flowed out of me at the moment I saw her gave me all the strength I needed to cope with our – and more particularly her – tribulations that followed: the heart operation that led to the brain damage that led to her being epileptic, blind and so profoundly handicapped she could do very little for herself for the eight years of her life. But I always felt equal to the task of helping her live each day because of this free flow of loving energy, over which I had no control whatsoever. If that flow had been blocked, if for some reason I hadn't connected with this baby, I am fairly sure I would have been defeated very early on. And then I dread to think what would have happened.

The free flow of emotional energy is of the most vital importance.

Robert Becker MD, author of the book *Cross Currents*, tells the story of two men of about the same age who both developed leukaemia at about the same time – and both consulted the same doctor. One of them submitted to the prescribed course of chemotherapy uncomplainingly, while the other refused to have anything to do with it. The doctor asked the willing patient to 'counsel' the other man in order to persuade him to take the chemo but the latter refused point blank. This second patient was an angry man who responded to the situation by going into rages, often smashing plates and glasses against the walls of his house. The good patient endured the first course of chemo and when that failed underwent a further treatment with an experimental drug, and when that failed he died after two years. Becker was writing more than ten years after this event. The bad patient was at that time still alive.

The bad patient, we should note, gave full vent to his angers. It may not have been pretty to watch but it was free flowing. It is not anger so much as bottled up anger that is lethal. And of course we don't know what else this bad patient did – the things he didn't tell his doctor about.

But many people with cancer do not feel such intense anger – indeed, as Lawrence LeShan pointed out, many people with cancer feel divorced not only from positive emotions, they are also divorced from negative ones. As one of his patients told him: 'It's not that I've been or done anything. It's that I've done nothing and been nothing.'

One of LeShan's patients was a lawyer who was married to a wife for whom he was a trophy husband. However, 'John', as he refers to him, actually wanted to be a musician. Eventually, having gone through counselling, he found in himself the confidence to go for it. He gave up his job, divorced his wife and trained to be a classical musician, eventually getting a job with an orchestra – and his terminal brain cancer disappeared.

Pattie, another cancer patient, told me personally of how cancer made her re-evaluate her life: 'This experience changed my entire life – body, soul and spirit. I am a new woman. I changed my diet, quit my stressful job, sold my too-big house, rid myself of all negative friends, and divorced my alcoholic hubby.' The result? 'I had no idea what real happiness was until 2002.'

So what can we learn from all this?

The first thing we can learn is that love – and happiness is an expression of love – is a powerful, all conquering emotion. Our goal is to attain it or allow it to flow through us. Sometimes love just happens, but sometimes we have to work at it. One way of harnessing the power of love is to get rid of the obstacles to love that are in the way: the too-big house, the alcoholic hubby, the wrong job, or whatever it is.

Another thing we can do is to get rid of all the anger we have harboured. Think about all the people that you feel anger or hatred for. Now forgive them. That's right. As you bring each one to mind, enter fully into a state of forgiveness. You don't need to reconcile with these people and you don't need to understand why they did whatever it was they did; you just need to be at peace with them. Let the hatred and anger go. Give them your whole-hearted blessing.

It may be that the person you feel most anger and upset at is yourself. LeShan had an exercise that helped. For each incident or moment that inspired anger or self-hatred, LeShan suggested that in your mind's eye you go back to talk to the person you once were and tell them that you love them. Just that. Love, embrace and, above all, forgive yourself.

Counselling, or any form of psychotherapy, can of course be immensely helpful. So too can art therapy – or indeed just letting yourself engage with any form of creative endeavour. This will allow subconscious themes to emerge, which you may focus on or not as you wish. Spending time in nature can also help engage the healing powers of the contemplative mind. Indeed, in times long gone, hugging trees and breathing in the fumes of organic soils were considered to be curative – and science has shown soil to have health promoting qualities due to the mix of microorganisms it contains.

Taking up a sport, going away for a holiday to some place

you've always wanted to visit: these may be seen by others as a form of escapism but you should see it as fulfilling a dream. And why should your dreams not be fulfilled? Perhaps what you really need to do is to climb Mount Everest, or go to Paris for a year to learn French, or take up sailing, or work as a volunteer in a home for the handicapped in Calcutta. Only you can know what it would please your heart to do.

As you get to know your past and present emotional conditioning, over time you will see all the unhelpful mental states and attitudes that have contributed to creating your illness. And as you become aware of your negative tendencies, it will become easier to let them go or change them into positive, health-supporting habits of mind.

Christopher Sheppard

In November 1999, Christopher Sheppard, a film producer, was diagnosed with 'locally advanced' rectal cancer and his doctors recommended surgery — as did the homoeopathic doctors and acupuncturist that he approached to help him. However, Sheppard refused surgery and chemo. But eventually, after a lot of soul searching, he did decide to accept radiation treatment. He also decided to go on what he called a healing journey. It was his view that each cancer victim, not their doctor, should be the authority on what they should do for their cancer. And they should make their decisions on the basis of their own self-knowledge, intuition and sense of the world.

For himself, he selected a modified version of the Gerson diet, developed by his nutritionist, heavily supplemented with vitamins, minerals and herbs. At one point he was taking over a hundred pills a day.

He also decided to visit a Brazilian spiritual healer, Joao Texeira, also known to his followers as 'John of God'. He felt strongly that there was a spiritual dimension, that his cancer was a sign of a spiritual malaise. This led him to Tibetan Buddhism and he studied a special form of meditation at a Buddhist community. Another self-devised therapy was to join an emotional counselling group.

Within a year he was cancer free and remains so to this day. Radiation on its own is not generally considered curative for rectal cancers.

Christopher describes his journey in great detail at his website at *www.christopher-sheppard.com*.

Relax and Laugh

Relax and laugh? This may seem a strategy too far. I can imagine you shouting: How the hell can you tell me to relax and laugh when I've been told I've got cancer?

For many years *Reader's Digest* has run a joke section called 'Laughter's the Best Medicine'. And, indeed, it may very well be one of nature's finest medicines. The classic study of the benefit of laughter was undertaken by Norman Cousins using himself as a guinea pig. In his book *An Anatomy of an Illness as Perceived by the Patient* he described how he fell victim to a devastating metabolic condition that the doctors could do nothing to cure. Cousins booked himself out of hospital and into a hotel room. He then set up a film projector and screen and began to watch one comedy film after another: Chaplin, the Marx Brothers, Buster Keaton and everyone else he found amusing. His theory was very simple. If bad emotions have bad effects on the body, wouldn't that mean that good emotions — love, hope, faith, laughter and confidence — would have a good effect on the body?

There is a simple, non-specific test that measures overall health of the body. This is the blood sedimentation test which measures how quickly or slowly red blood cells settle to the bottom of a test tube (the 'sed rate' as it is known). The faster they settle, the higher the sed rate, the worse the overall state of health is. Cousins discovered that he could get real pain relief and cumulative improvements in the sed rate through laughter. The benefits of laughter were, he discovered, measurable using the sed rate test. This means that having fun is good for you. Norman Cousins didn't have cancer but the truth he discovered is as true for cancer as the ailment that afflicted him – and from which he eventually recovered.

So, get out those old comedies, knockabout farces, slapstick routines – whatever it takes to get you laughing. Of all the positive emotions that Cousins listed, laughter is the only one with a strong physiological element. It provides a real and immediate release of stress and anxiety.

Let's now turn our attention from laughter to stress and anxiety.

It is now known that stress is not just a cause of illness but that it makes cancers more aggressive. Relaxation – the complete absence of stress – on the other hand is healing. Some people have been told that there is no cure for their cancer. They have gone home and recovered simply because they accepted their fate and found themselves valued and nurtured by their loved ones. They were happy and their happiness helped them to heal themselves. A Japanese study into cases of spontaneous healing found that this was almost always associated with a feeling of complete acceptance of their situation.

It is for this reason that those who grimly mutter 'I will get better. I will get better' are unlikely to achieve their goal. You can almost feel the anxiety and stress in their determined positivity. The goal is to let go, to accept, to embrace, in short, to relax completely.

One of the problems with being diagnosed with cancer is that this induces enormous anxiety and stress. This in turn has the unfortunate effect of making a cancer more aggressive. It is therefore important to do whatever one can to reduce anxiety.

One strategy is denial. Some people have been known to be so unable to deal with the problem that they have quite simply decided to forget about it. Interestingly, 'going into denial' – as this is sometimes referred to – can be a successful strategy. Some people have lived with their cancer for a very long time, and indeed, if some anecdotal reports are to be trusted, have even cured themselves – simply by ignoring it. However, since denial is an absence of conscious attention, it is not one that can be advocated in a book like this. Also, we need to recognize that the term 'denial' is a difficult one to deal with. From the outside it may appear that someone is denying reality, while to the person involved, a very different psychological process is being experienced. Perhaps the person just doesn't trust others sufficiently to be honest about it.

If you are caring for someone who has gone into denial, one important potential benefit needs to be borne in mind.

One medical statistician, Dr Hardin Jones, calculated in the 1960s that people who did nothing for their cancers were on average likely to live four times longer than those who did something. 'Doing something' in this case meant undergoing one or more of the orthodox treatments. Treatments have improved very little since that time, so this conclusion remains as relevant today as it was then. So the person who is 'in denial' is at least not subjecting themselves to burdensome, life-shortening treatments. However, I don't wish to appear to be advocating denial as a strategy. A state of awareness and relaxed acceptance of the situation must surely be preferable.

There are many ways of inducing relaxation. Sunbathing is one. The warm rays of the sun really do induce healing — forget all that anti-sun propaganda. The sun doesn't just relax you. It helps you absorb vitamin D, which, as we shall see later, is itself a powerful cancer fighter. All sunblocks — organic or otherwise — interfere with the production of vitamin D. Of course it's not a good idea to get burnt, but if you are sensible that won't happen. Sunblocks packed with artificial chemicals are not to be recommended. However there are increasing numbers of organic sunblocks coming onto the market. But the ideal is to let unprotected skin be exposed to the sun for, say, half an hour in the tropics — much longer at more northerly climes. If you do happen to get burnt then a quick application of aloe vera gel and lavender essential oil will quickly heal the burnt skin.

One other point needs to be made. It is common to read warnings that you need to protect your eyes with sunglasses when out in the strong sunlight because of an increased risk of getting cataracts. This is true, but cataracts are easy to treat and there is good reason for not wearing sunglasses. The light that enters the eyes stimulates the endocrine and pineal glands. Light is a nutrient, and we eat its benefits as much through the eyes as through the skin. Glasses interfere with this, so dispense with them for as long as you can. Even untinted glasses should be dispensed with when outdoors.

Other means of enhancing laughter and relaxation whilst reducing stress and anxiety are all forms of sport, exercise, meditation, and listening to certain types of music. (My favourites are Javanese gamelan or Indian dulcimer – santoor – music, and I do heartily recommend the music of Shiv Kumar Sharma.) Reading the works of P.G. Wodehouse or James Thurber or any other comic writer is also beneficial. In short, involve yourself with whoever or whatever can raise a smile or any other feeling of wholehearted pleasure.

For those who need a chemical aid to eliminate anxiety, the amino acid L-theanine comes highly recommended. This is a key ingredient of green tea leaves but is available and best taken as a purified extract. Make sure this is in the form Suntheanine which is a patented pharmaceutical grade L-theanine from Japan.

Lastly, a word about the importance of sleep. It is extremely important to get as much sleep as you can. Eight hours a night is recommended. It is also recommended that you sleep in a completely dark room. The reason for this is that melatonin, a hormone secreted by the pineal gland, plays a very important role in healing. It is known that people who work nights have a higher incidence of illness – including cancer. Our own melatonin production falls as we grow older. Light interferes with the secretion of melatonin. Poor sleepers may consider supplementing with melatonin. Other natural sleep aids that I have found useful are valerian herb, St John's wort herb and that most wonderful of all healing agents, organic lavender essential oil. Vetiver essential oil is also a wonderful relaxant.

So, to summarize the key points of the first four strategies: be nice to yourself, eliminate negativity, relax, laugh, free the power of the emotions and harness the power of the imaginative mental image. And you don't have to be too heroic – just keep accumulating small achievements.

Michael Gearin-Tosh

Michael Gearin-Tosh was, for 35 years, tutor in English at St Catherine's College, Oxford. In 1994 he was diagnosed with myeloma, a cancer of the bone marrow. Although urged to take chemotherapy, he discovered that this would give him only a 4% possibility of a cure. His conclusion: 'Touch it [chemo], and you're a goner.'

He embarked on a series of alternative treatments consisting of twelve freshly made vegetable juices a day, high-dose vitamin injections, acupuncture, raw garlic, coffee enemas and Chinese breathing exercises. He also used visualization techniques in which he imagined his immune cells attacking the tumour. The result was that his cancer went into remission. He was still cancer free eleven years later when he died in 2005 from an untreated blood infection.

Gearin-Tosh described his battle with cancer in his book *Living Proof, A Medical Mutiny* (2002).

Strategy 5:

Detox the Body

In Strategies 1–4 we looked at the very 'soft', but no less important, areas of bringing our thoughts, emotions and mental processes into a state of readiness to engage full-heartedly and full-mindedly with whatever it is we choose to do in order to recover completely and permanently from cancer.

We must now turn our attention to the body as a whole, to see in what ways we can return it to a state of health. But first let us visualize a scenario. Let us imagine that the strategy we have chosen is successfully attacking a cancer tumour. The result may be that the cancer tumour starts to die and dis-integrate. Obviously the body needs to deal with this poisonous waste. It needs to eliminate it just as it eliminates everything else. But, if we have cancer, almost certainly there will be some form of pre-existing toxicity in the colon. And the liver, whose job is to detoxify poisons, will be in a weakened state. We will therefore be adding a toxic burden to organs that are not yet fit to deal with them. The result is that the poisons will be reabsorbed into the body and we will feel worse. This situation is called the Herxheimer response. If this happens – and we must read our body sensitively at all times to see how it is coping with the therapies we are undertaking – then it is a good idea to desist for a day or two until symptoms ease and we can continue.

So, before we do anything else, we need to pay attention to detoxifying the body. The first element of detoxification must be to stop putting more poisons into the body. That means paying attention to the food and drink we are taking in. Meat, dairy products, sugar and alcohol should be completely eliminated from our diet and replaced by raw (or steamed) vegetables and fruit. Steaming, unlike other ways of cooking food, does not deplete the vitamin and mineral content – or very much less so than other ways of cooking. The only drink we should allow ourselves at first is water and we should drink as much water as we can tolerate – say 10 to 15 glasses a day. There are one or two specialized waters that you may want to consider: Willard water, alkaline electrolysed water and even distilled water are recommended. However, plain ordinary tap water is better than nothing. Exceptions to this regime can be made for certain teas: peppermint, sage, ginger or green tea. Additionally, freshly made carrot and beetroot juices are particularly healthy for the liver. Adding some fresh lemon juice to the water is also beneficial.

Of course a diet that consists exclusively of raw fruit and vegetables will be naturally detoxifying over time and no other special methods may be necessary.

This is the first step in our detoxification programme.

Now that we have dealt with the input, we need to look at

the output. Colon cleansing is where to start. There are various strategies for doing this. Firstly we can undergo a series of colonic irrigations. There are some cautions, however; it is not a good idea if you have a colon cancer or a number of other conditions (and certainly not if you're pregnant). If a full colonic is not possible, then it is a good idea to take a good dose of magnesium oxide in a glass of water. This should induce a speedy elimination of impacted faecal material. You may also consider taking bentonite clay, a good charcoal powder (one that does not contain sugar) and/or psyllium husks. All of these bind with toxins and help clear the intestines.

Now that we have cleaned the colon we can turn our attention to the liver. Some people advocate a liver cleanse to flush out toxins. However, if the liver itself is cancerous this may not be advisable. It may be better to simply support the liver in less drastic ways. I have already mentioned the benefits of carrot and beetroot juice. The liver can also be supported by taking a regular supplement of the following herbs: rosemary, milk thistle and dandelion root. Vitamin C, lemon juice and apple cider vinegar are also very supportive for the liver.

One method for detoxing the liver is to give yourself a coffee retention enema. The coffee is drawn up into the rectum and held for as long as possible. It draws poisons out and flushes them out. You can buy coffee specially designed for this purpose as well as equipment and instructions via the internet. (A simple search for 'coffee enema' will lead you to a number of helpful sites.) Alternatively, instead of coffee, flaxseed oil can be used for the retention enema with the same results. Retention enemas are particularly useful if you are feeling nauseous, which is an indication that the liver is being overloaded with toxins.

Then there is the lymph system. A very light lymphatic massage may be helpful. The object of a lymphatic massage is to get the lymph moving. Another way, indeed possibly the best way, is to get a rebounder – a small personal trampoline – and to bounce or jog on it gently for up to 45 minutes a day (while watching TV perhaps). You may find that, to start with, just doing 5 minutes may give you more exercise than your leg muscles are used to.

The skin is another important organ of elimination. Skin brushing should be done with a long handled bristle brush made of natural materials. The skin should be dry, not wet, when brushed. Some practitioners recommend that the abdomen should be brushed in an anticlockwise direction and other areas should be brushed towards the heart. Brush each part of the body several times vigorously – though breasts should be brushed lightly, avoiding the nipples which should not be brushed at all. Start with the soles of the feet because the nerve endings there affect the whole body, then the ankles, calves and thighs, up across your buttocks, stomach and chest. After the brushing session you can have a shower.

Lying in a warm bath in which Dead Sea salt (or Himalayan salt) has been dissolved is very detoxing – as is a lengthy time spent in the sea.

Then there are traditional saunas, infrared lamp saunas, steam rooms and ionizing footbaths. All of these are helpful for the detoxification process – especially the ionizing foot-baths. It might be worth considering buying one. While some ionizing footbaths are quite expensive, there are a number of cheaper products on the market made in China or Indonesia.

It is a sad truth that we live in an environment heavily polluted by toxic chemicals. Even polar bears, who live in one of the remotest habitats on earth, have been found to be contaminated with DDT. Each and every one of us contains toxic residues of these chemicals which have an impact on our health. We cannot hope to avoid this contamination but we can do what we can to eliminate it as quickly from our bodies as possible through a process known as chelation. There are a number of natural chelating agents. Vitamin C is one, the chemical EDTA is another. An internet search will locate a number of commercial oral chelation products that you might wish to consider. Some clinics offer intravenous chelation.

Another product that claims to aid cellular health in a number of ways, including detoxification and chelation, is PolyMVA (the initials stand for Minerals, Vitamins and Amino acids). This is a patented formulation in which the element palladium has been complexed with alpha lipoic acid

and a number of other vitamins and minerals. It is claimed
that this substance is a powerful re-energizer of cells, immune
stimulant, chelator of heavy metals, detoxifier, and that it
helps maintain alkaline pH levels. There are a number of
convincing testimonials relating to the benefits of PolyMVA
for a wide range of cancers both on its own or as part of a
parcel of alternative therapies. The only problem with Poly-
MVA is the price: it is fairly expensive! For further information go to *www.polymva.org*.

In addition, the following herbs may be helpful for detoxifying and cleansing the following organs and systems:

Herb	Benefits
burdock root	liver, blood, skin
cascara sagrada	natural laxative
cayenne pepper	digestive system, blood
dandelion root	digestive system, liver, diuretic
echinacea	lymph, anti-viral, immune system stimulant
fennel	mild laxative
garlic	blood, digestive system
ginger root	circulation
liquorice root	hormone balancer
goldenseal	blood, liver, kidney, skin
Oregon grape	blood, colon, liver, skin
parsley leaf	diuretic
red clover	blood, glands, immune system

So, to conclude, a week or two of detoxification makes sense, before starting in earnest on the other strategies – both those focused on the whole body and those aimed at the cancer itself.

Fred Eichhorn

In 1976, Fred was found to have islet cell carcinoma and was given a maximum life expectancy of three years, though most of the doctors he consulted believed he would be dead within a year. He underwent surgery in which 90% of his pancreas was removed along with his spleen and part of his stomach. However, this was not expected to provide a cure. Fred decided to define the problem. He felt that in every case ill health follows like a domino effect from a first cause. The solution is to find that first cause in terms of the body's biochemistry and correct it. Then a good domino effect will result in the elimination of the disease.

He decided good nutrition – a return to pre-1900s standards, i.e. completely organic – along with exercise and a positive mental framework were the cornerstones of good health.

In 1980 Fred enrolled in medical college and studied for four years followed by a further three years' research.

Fred Eichhorn is cancer free today 30 years later, and so committed is he to spreading the word that he has set up the National Cancer Research Foundation (*www.ncrf.org*) and offers help and information completely free of charge. He provides a number of testimonials on his site of people who have benefited from following his regime.

Strategy 6:

Oxidize the Body

We now know that the cause of the vast majority, if not all, cancers is the low oxygenation of the surrounding tissues. This low oxygen state forces some cells to find a different way to satisfy their energy needs. They can no longer get adequate energy supplies using the normal aerobic channels, so they change over to a primitive anaerobic mode of energy production, similar to fermentation.

One of the first things to happen as the cell converts from one state to the other is that the cell switches off the mitochondria, which are rodlike structures in the cell whose job is to provide energy through aerobic means. Unfortunately, shutting down the mitochondria has a further deleterious effect: the cell can no longer trigger its own death (because this is another function mediated by the mitochondria). It therefore, in effect, becomes immortal — which is why cancer is a real problem. Cancer cells replicate themselves but cannot trigger their own death so, if nothing else changes the situation, they grow and grow, eventually taking over the entire system.

One way to change the situation is to increase the tissue oxygen levels of the entire body. This will have the effect of persuading the cells to change back to a normal state by switching the mitochondria back on. As soon as this happens the cell will trigger its own death and the cancer tumour will die. That at least is the theory and it is supported by a great deal of laboratory research. There are also personal testimonials from people who have followed an oxygen-enhancing therapy and gone on to live long lives free of cancer. Take Cliff Beckwith, a retired educationalist living near Knoxville, Tennessee. In 1991 he was diagnosed with stage 4 prostate cancer, which means that the cancer had spread widely. He was not expected to live long. He eventually died in 2007. He lived to a ripe old age, mostly free from cancer, because he followed one of the therapies below.

So, how can we enhance the oxygenation of the body's tissues?

Oxygen and ozone

One way is to take in oxygen directly. At first sight it might appear that this can be done by breathing oxygen in from a canister. Such canisters are marketed on the internet and they claim to help people to improve their health in a number of ways. However, there is only so much pure oxygen that we can breathe in without causing oxygen toxicity. So trying to solve your oxygenation needs in this way is not recommended, although a little-but-often approach might be a useful addition to other approaches.

Another way is to undergo some form of ozonating therapy.

Ozone (O_3) is unstable and quickly changes to oxygen (O_2). There are clinics in Germany and Mexico which offer a form of ozone therapy in which blood is drawn from the patient, passed through an ozonating machine and then reintroduced to the body. However, a less expensive and more convenient way of introducing ozone into the body is to get an ozone generating machine and to bubble ozone through water (this, by the way, quickly sterilizes the water). In some countries, swimming pools are maintained using ozone generators rather than chlorine. Since chlorine is a poison while ozone isn't, the superiority of this approach is evident. Swimming pool operators please note!

Hydrogen peroxide

Some people advocate increasing the body's oxygen levels by means of hydrogen peroxide. Hydrogen peroxide can be taken in many ways. Doctors prefer to give it in the form of an intravenous drip, and this is probably the best way when chronic illness is being treated. However, it can be taken at home in other ways. But it is important to note that hydrogen peroxide in strengths greater than 3% is dangerous. It can normally be bought in strengths of 3% or 6% from any chemist shop. Food grade hydrogen peroxide is 35%. This is the purest form and many advocates of hydrogen peroxide therapy urge users to use food grade H_2O_2 for internal use. But it must be diluted! Undiluted H_2O_2 is extremely dangerous. A drop of food grade H_2O_2 on the skin will cause a white burn mark. Anyone with children should not have it around the house!

Hydrogen peroxide can be taken orally, it can be added to a bath, it can be rubbed on the skin, or it can be gargled as a mouthwash. *Suggested quantities are as follows.*

For oral use – either for drinking or mouthwash:
35% food grade: increasing daily from 1 drop to 25 drops in a glass of water. However, it appears that not many people can tolerate 25 drops in a glass of water.
6% solution: $\frac{1}{2}$ a teaspoon to 2 teaspoons in an 8-ounce glass of water.
Double this for 3% solution.

Physical activity

But we don't have to take oxygen directly in the form of oxygen, ozone or hydrogen peroxide in order to increase tissue oxygen levels. We can simply go for a stiff walk, a light jog, a swim. Or we can do a light form of exercise that will move the upper body: T'ai Chi or Qigong are particularly recommended. Indeed there is a form of Qigong that was specifically developed as a cancer therapy and there is a growing movement in Beijing where it is taught in some of that city's parks. Ms Guo Lin, a Chinese traditional painter, was originally diagnosed with cancer of the uterus in 1949. It was surgically removed but the cancer recurred in 1960 and she was told that her condition was terminal. At this point she remembered that her grandfather had taught her as a child to practise Qigong. She studied his books and created her own system of Qigong exercise. She practised this form of Qigong for two hours every day, and six months later tests showed that her cancer had shrunk.

She continued her practice and eventually, in 1970, she started giving lessons in a Beijing park in what she called New Qigong Therapy. By 1977 she felt she had demonstrated clearly that Qigong had been beneficial for many cancer patients and she announced publicly that Qigong could cure cancer. Her fame spread and soon, everyday, she was leading three to four hundred people through their Qigong paces. She became a national celebrity, travelling around China to demonstrate her system. Although she died in 1984, her system of Qigong is still widely practised.

So, exercise is another way to enhance the oxygen levels of the body.

The Budwig protocol

Finally, there is one more oxygen-enhancing approach that adherents claim can help cure 90% of cancers. This figure is of course speculative as the approach has not been subjected to the scrutiny of randomized clinical trials (but the fault for that lies firmly with the public bodies whose job it is to oversee medical research). This is the therapy that Cliff Beckwith, whose story I mentioned at the start of this chapter, followed.

Dr Johanna Budwig was one of the pioneering scientists who first studied fats. She soon realized that some fats were extremely beneficial for our health. She eventually developed what is now known as the Budwig protocol – a health plan that claims not only to cure cancer but also arthritis and heart disease as well.

For oxygen to reach all parts of the body it must be carried there in the haemoglobin of the blood. If the haemoglobin is in a depleted or unhealthy state it cannot carry the oxygen to where it is needed. Omega 3 oils are needed to maintain the haemoglobin in a healthy state. Johanna Budwig saw that although fish oils are a more available source of omega 3 oils, they nevertheless require processing by the liver. However, she saw that there was a way of harnessing the omega 3 oils in flaxseeds, which are normally less bio-available, while at the same time bypassing the liver (it is important to bypass the liver because it will almost certainly be in a diseased state). She argued that dissolving the omega 3 oils in flaxseeds by thoroughly blending them – by hand, with a spoon – with a sulphur-based protein (either quark or low-fat cottage cheese) would result in the flaxseed oil becoming water soluble and so easily absorbed into the body without having to go via the liver. For people with cancer she proposed that they should take a tablespoonful of organic liquid flaxseed oil (not capsules!) six times a day. The oil should be standard – not in any way 'enhanced' (some brands market a 'high-lignan' oil, which should be avoided). It should be mixed with one or two tablespoons of quark or cottage cheese, a little cayenne pepper or garlic added if desired, and eaten. This is the simple core of her protocol. It should be accompanied by a diet that is largely vegetarian and by lengthy spells of exposure to sunlight. For more precise details and testimonials, I recommend that you go to the flaxseedoil2 yahoo discussion group, which Cliff Beckwith nurtured in its early days. One important caution when following this protocol is to avoid all other forms of supplement, especially antioxidant supplements such as vitamin C as they interfere with its effectiveness.

As I say, Johanna Budwig claims that six spoons of flaxseed oil taken this way is curative. And if it isn't, then increase the daily consumption to ten spoons a day. There are many testimonials supporting its effectiveness − even in the case of brain cancers. It should also be noted that flaxseeds are very rich in lignans, a group of plant-based chemicals that experiments have shown to be powerful anti-cancer agents in their own right.

Cliff Beckwith

Cliff Beckwith, a retired educationalist living near Knoxville, Tennessee, was one of the founders of the Yahoo health group's information resource on flaxseed oil. Here he tells his own story:

'In January 1991 I was diagnosed with advanced prostate cancer. Bone scans and other tests indicated no spread so it was decided to operate. During the operation it was discovered that the cancer had spread to the lymph glands, making it stage four. The operation was not completed as that would not be the answer. The only treatment used was Lupron and Eulexin to cancel the male hormones. I was told the male hormone does not cause cancer, but if cancer is present it is like throwing kerosene on a fire.

'At the time of the attempted operation my PSA count was 75. It was six months before I had the second PSA. When the call came from the doctor's office I was told "Mr Beckwith! Your count is completely normal!" It was 0.1 and 0.1 to 0.4 is normal.

'The reason it was normal was because, in addition to the hormone drugs, I had started taking flaxseed oil mixed with cottage cheese. I had read a number of books recommending this approach, which was first formulated by Dr Johanna Budwig and is commonly known as the Budwig protocol.

'I quit Lupron after 4 years and 7 months in October of 1995 as it was no longer useful. I thought I was cured but not so. In roughly two years the PSA was again rising. I began changing the amounts I took of flaxseed oil/cottage cheese that led to a series of ups and downs with the PSA results.

'I learned that there are 30 strains of prostate cancer. They are all different and any man may have any combination of strains. This makes the problem different from individual to individual. Mine is a medium aggressive cancer.

'In January 2004 my PSA was 6.7, that is very close to normal for a man of 85. I thought I had it beaten. It had now been 13 years since diagnosis. Most men with advanced prostate cancer do not live nearly that long. The doctor told me after a couple of years that I was one of the lucky ones. Most men with the condition I had did not make it 6 months.

'In Jan. 2004 I decided to try ellagic acid, which has proved effective in many cases. However, my PSA went up instead of further down. Then I added lycopene. I had been told that it needed to be used heavily to be effective; three 12-ounce glasses of tomato juice a day. I did that for four months.

'Then I learned two things a couple of days apart. One was that Dr Budwig had said in 1956 that if one is using flaxseed oil one must not use heavy amounts of antioxidants as it would neutralize the effect of the flaxseed oil. The other was that both ellagic acid and lycopene are powerful antioxidants.

'For over a year I was hurting the effect of the flaxseed oil/cottage cheese and for four months I was cancelling it completely. The result was that the cancer again began to develop and by the time I woke up to this fact, the PSA had gone to 131.

'I know that prostate cancer in the prostate does not kill. What kills is the cancer in the tissues to which it spreads. Flaxseed oil pretty much stops the spread. Until I went the antioxidant route it hadn't spread in 13 years. Now there are signs it has spread to the bone.

'So I immediately increased the flaxseed oil to 6 tablespoons a day and am using my rebounder (small trampoline). The result appears to be beneficial. I had been aware of an enlargement in the prostate gland and now it is getting smaller and urination is easier. I do not believe I am in danger any more.' (February 2006)

Cliff Beckwith died, aged 85, in 2007.

Alkalize the Body

'I gradually came to the basic conclusion that, in a body with normal metabolism, cancer cannot develop. The normalization of the damaged metabolism is therefore the essential aim of any therapy.' These are the words of the late Dr Max Gerson, a German doctor who escaped from Nazi Germany only to become a victim of the American medical authorities who objected to his cancer cure diet, largely because there was no money in it for them. (His daughter, carrying on his work, now runs a Gerson clinic in Mexico.)

For Gerson, if a body is truly healthy, cancer will not develop. But what does it mean for a body to be 'normalized', to be 'healthy'? Clearly it must mean more than simply feeling well, as many people feel perfectly well while cancer is growing inside them.

One of the key elements of true tissue health is that the tissue is properly oxygenated. We dealt with this point in the last chapter. The other key point is the degree of acidity or alkalinity that any tissue shows. A healthy state for any tissue is to be slightly alkaline. An unhealthy state is to be acidic. The degree of acidity or alkalinity is normally measured using a litmus paper, which records the pH value of a liquid. If the paper shows a level of 7, it is neutral. Below 7 is acidic and above 7 is alkaline. However, while it is easy to check the pH of urine or saliva, it isn't easy to test the pH of muscles. Also, it isn't very useful doing highly specific tests because the values will vary throughout the day.

It is important to note that there is a direct relationship between the level of oxygenation and the relative acidity of the body. A low oxygen state leads inevitably to an acidic state and vice versa.

It should also be noted that one further cause of acidity in a cancerous situation is that the cancer cell, when it gets its energy through the primitive anaerobic fermentation process, produces lactic acid which becomes a burden on the physical system and adds to its acidification. The lactic acid build-up interferes with the oxygenation of neighbouring cells. It is hard even for a healthy system to clear out this load of acidity. Anyone who does sports will know how long the 'stiffness' resulting from lactic acid build-up lasts.

So, in order to get well again, we need to find ways to return a body away from an acidic state back to a slightly alkaline state.

The first way must be through diet. A vegetarian diet, especially a raw food diet of fruits and vegetables, is alkaline. Meat and dairy products, on the other hand, are acidic. It may seem strange that a fruit such as an orange, packed as it is with citric acid, should be alkaline in its effects on the body. But it is. Almost certainly the reason why most cancer diets work is that they return the body to an alkaline state. Many such diets have been formulated – the Gerson diet, the macrobiotic diet, the Moerman diet, the Dries diet, and so on.

Dr Cornelis Moerman, a Dutch doctor who became interested in the subject of diets and cancer, first became involved when a man by the name of Leendert Brinkman came to him seeking his help. He had a stomach tumour which had spread to his groin and legs (i.e. it was stage 4). The doctors had given up on him. Moerman told him to eat as many oranges and lemons as he could. He ate them 'by the truckload until I was up to my eyes in vitamin C'. A year later he was free of tumours. He went on to live to the age of 90. It may have been the vitamin C – that certainly didn't hurt – but it was also almost certainly the more important alkalizing properties of citric acid that cured him. Citric acid also interferes with the glycolytic process that cancers use to transform sugars into energy.

Apple cider vinegar is also a very powerful alkalizer. Drunk diluted in water – just a teaspoonful or two in a glass – is very thirst quenching and brings the body quickly back into an alkaline state. It can also be splashed onto the surface of the skin. Although this can be slightly uncomfortable it is a good way of getting its benefits to the breasts, say, or the legs and arms which are remote from the digestive system. The most highly rated organic vinegar is made by Bragg's. They also have a special deal for people fighting cancer. Contact them at *www.bragg.com*.

'Supergreens' is a generic name for powders and drinks based on barley sprouts, chlorella or similar foods. Some will have up to 40 or more ingredients. These played a key part in Anne Frahm's cancer cure mentioned on page 29. Anne Frahm lived off a combination of green drinks, carrot juice and vitamin C, along with a few herbal drinks, for the duration of her ultimately successful five week cancer cure. I do recommend her book *Cancer Battle Plan*, which she co-wrote with her husband.

A teaspoon of sodium bicarbonate in a glass of water, taken last thing before bed, is also recommended as a way to increase alkalinity. Indeed, some go further and suggest that taking sodium bicarbonate throughout the day – and even intravenously – can be curative. It should, where possible, be introduced close to the site of the tumour, i.e. a vaginal flush may be helpful in the case of cervical cancer or by injection in the case of a breast cancer. However, taking it around meal times should be avoided as it will interfere with the stomach acids needed to digest foods.

An Italian doctor, Tullio Simoncini, bases his radical approach on the assumption that cancer is caused by fungus (specifically *Candida albicans*) and treats his patients, with seeming success, with 5% solution of sodium bicarbonate injected close to the site of the tumour. For more detailed discussion of his treatment go to *www.curenaturalicancro.com*.

Lying in the sun, among its many other benefits, also improves alkalinity.

Drinking alkaline ionized water is also highly recommended. This will require you to fit a special ionizing machine to your kitchen water outlet. There are a number of machines on the market and an internet search is recommended to locate one that is suitable. Remember that 70–80% of our bodies consists of water. Water is common to every tissue in our bodies. If we can make this water alkaline we will certainly be making our tissues alkaline as well.

Caesium chloride

Finally, for those who wish to consider a more extreme way of shifting the body to an alkaline state, there is a substance, cesium chloride, that does have a very powerful alkalizing effect. It will shift the body's tissues quickly to a pH level of 8, which is highly toxic for cancer cells. Caesium chloride also seems to work against cancer in other ways that are not fully understood. It is one of a few substances that are easily – and indeed preferentially – absorbed by cancer cells, but it cannot be eliminated from the same cell and so eventually kills the cell. The reason it is favoured by cancer cells is because it mimics potassium. But, precisely because of this feature, caesium can be dangerous in that it can lead to potassium deprivation. Potassium supplementation is vital, but it also needs to be carefully monitored. Too little potassium is very dangerous (for the healthy operation of the heart among other things), but so is too much. Generally speaking, supplementing with about 3 grams a day in divided doses should be about right for an average individual. But since people vary enormously in terms of size and weight, you should consult with your doctor on how your potassium needs can be monitored. However, with this proviso, caesium does appear to be a relatively safe, inexpensive and effective treatment, which if taken under close medical supervision can be effective in killing cancer or slowing down the speed of its development.

Very importantly, caesium chloride also neutralizes the toxic breakdown products released when a cancer tumour starts to die off. This means that cesium would be a useful accompaniment to any therapy deemed to be effective, as it is not unknown for some patients to die because the anti-cancer therapy they were following was too effective. They died from the toxicity of the cancer as it haemorrhaged.

The proposed dose of caesium is a minimum of 3 grams a day (less than this can have the reverse effect of promoting tumour growth), but 6–10 grams a day is better (don't worry, toxic levels are well over 100 grams a day). It should be taken with vitamin C (5–10 grams), vitamin A (100,000 iu), zinc (50–100 mg) and potassium (3 grams). Magnesium (1 gram) is also useful as this mineral mediates the sodium-potassium balance. These supplements must be continued for at least three months after use of caesium has been discontinued, as it stays in the body depleting potassium levels for that length of time.

Side effects that might be experienced are some nausea, diarrhoea, sweating, tingling around the lips, and there may be some problem relating to an excess of uric acid. Also of course there will be the effects of the cancer tumour breaking up. These will depend on where the tumour is and how well the body can deal with it, but may include flu-like symptoms.

Dr Keith Brewer, who first promoted the use of cesium chloride in the 1970s and 80s, also recommended that caesium could be usefully combined with laetrile (see page 136) as this will help minimize side effects and, at the same time, promote its effectiveness.

Caesium chloride is cheaply available on the internet. One source that has useful information is *www.rainbowminerals.net.*

Why isn't this therapy undertaken in hospitals? Because it is 'unproven'. Why is it unproven? Because it hasn't been put through the kind of large scale, randomized clinical trials that alone can prove or disprove the value of a therapy. And why hasn't it? Good question.

Beata Bishop

Beata Bishop was panic-stricken when a mole on her leg was diagnosed as melanoma, one of the fastest spreading and most lethal of all cancers. She underwent painful and disfiguring surgery but within a year it was found that the cancer had spread into the lymphatic system. Rather than undergo further extensive surgery she chose instead to follow the diet developed by an eminent German physician, Dr Max Gerson. Taking her fate in her hands, she spent two months at the world's only Gerson clinic in Mexico where she learnt the theory and practice of the intensive therapy, which she then pursued for a further 18 months in London.

After two years on the Gerson Therapy, which transformed her both physically and psychologically, Beata Bishop made a full recovery. Today, in her 70s, she is still alive, extremely active and free of her cancer. She wrote her story in a book, *My Triumph Over Cancer*, first published in 1985.

Strategy 8:

Empower the Body

The body has a number of defence systems that protect it from attack by viruses, bacteria, fungi and other parasitic infestations. It also has ways of healing itself when it receives an injury which needs to be repaired. These are extraordinarily complex responses which are constantly evolving to respond to threats which are also evolving. We refer to all these diverse ways of responding to threats from the outside as the immune system.

One big question for scientists is why our bodies don't attack cancer tumours. Tumours are clearly a threat to the system. Why are they not responded to as viruses and bacteria are responded to, i.e. as soon as they are detected? Instead they are allowed to grow and spread throughout the system without triggering an immune response. What's going on and what can we do about it?

One obvious answer is that the body doesn't react to a tumour because a tumour is not a foreign body. It is composed of the body's own cells. However, the body's immune system can be triggered to attack cancer tumours. And the body's immune system can, in addition, be strengthened to such an extent that the cancer tumour is unable to spread and grow – at worst the tumour progression is slowed down. At best, it is put into reverse.

So, in what ways can we boost the immune system?

Vitamin C

The famous biochemist Linus Pauling and a Scottish doctor Ewan Cameron formulated the theory that cancer could be impeded by strengthening the collagen material that surrounds each cell. This would prevent cancer from invading new tissues. The key element needed to achieve this aim was vitamin C.

Vitamin C is a very important substance and humans, primates and – interestingly – the guinea pig are among the very few mammals that need to get their vitamin C from food. It is believed that our ancestors succumbed to a genetic disease that killed off the enzyme that in most mammals produces the vitamin C in their livers. And those animals that produce vitamin C produce lots of it. These high levels of production appear to lead to the conclusion that a 'normal' level of intake of vitamin C for human beings would be in the region of 8–12 grams a day – and that's on a nice sunny day when we're feeling pretty good. On a bad day, when we're cold, wet and miserable and battling with bacteria and viruses – or cancer – we might need 50–100 grams, or even more. These are the figures that animal studies indicate are reasonable. This is supported by another fact. When we take in vitamin C it is impossible to get an overdose. First it is entirely non-toxic in its effects, but if the body takes in more than it can handle it dumps the surplus by provoking diarrhoea. The amount needed to provoke this response is known as the bowel tolerance level. And again we get the same sort of figures. To produce this result on a good day it will probably take 8–12 grams, and on a bad day 60 or more grams. The bowel tolerance level is therefore a very accurate method to determine the vitamin C needs of the body. In the case of cancer, it is likely to be in the area of 30–50 grams a day. So we can conclude that, optimally, we should be taking in a level of vitamin C that is just a little below the bowel tolerance level.

Now most people are familiar with vitamin C in the form of bright orange tablets that effervesce as they dissolve in a glass of water. This is probably the worst possible way of taking vitamin C. The commonly available calcium ascorbate and forms of vitamin C such as Ester-C are not recommended as some consider them not to be effective. Best is to buy, in powder or crystal form, either L-ascorbic acid or the non-acidic sodium ascorbate salt. Bronson's is one highly regarded source – it is the one that Linus Pauling himself used (see *www.bronsonvitamins.com*) – but there are many other perfectly acceptable products. When taking vitamin C orally care should be taken to build up intake slowly – by say 1–2 grams a day – to the desired level.

It is also possible to take vitamin C in much higher doses,

100–150 grams a day, intravenously. In this case only the sodium ascorbate form is suitable. You will need to find a doctor or clinic willing to do this for you. The following web page gives some useful advice: *www.doctoryourself.com/ strategies.*

Dr Matthias Rath, a follower of Linus Pauling, has suggested that large doses of vitamin C (10–30 grams) should be accompanied by equally large doses of the amino acid L-lysine and half that amount of L-proline, both of which help protect against collagen dissolving enzymes. For further details you can download his free book at *www.dr-rath-foundation.org.*

Finally, a newly developed form of vitamin C, Lypo-Spheric vitamin C, claims to be far more bio-available than other forms so that very little is 'wasted' in urine. For more information go to *www.livonlabs.com.* I have read a number of testimonials in free discussion groups of how easy this form of vitamin C is to tolerate and how quickly it has an effect. It may be that if the claims are true, that 100% of the vitamin C gets through to the cells, then Lypo-Spheric vitamin C taken orally would have the same impact as vitamin C taken intravenously.

In addition to vitamin C there are a number of other powerful immune system stimulants.

Agaricus blazei Murill

This is a Brazilian mushroom, also known as ABM, that has demonstrated remarkable anti-cancer properties. Normally, the polysaccharides found in fungus only affect solid cancers, but the class of polysaccharides in *Agaricus blazei* is effective against almost all cancers. In one Japanese study, ABM was found to eliminate all cancerous tumours in 90% of the experimental mice. In another study the mice were fed *Agaricus blazei* as a preventative and then injected with a very powerful cancer-causing agent; 99.4% of them showed no tumour growth.

In the case of serious illness, take 40 grams a day (about 2 mushrooms) and simmer for an hour in water (at a ratio of one litre per mushroom). Taking vitamin C promotes absorption. Agaricus and other mushrooms can be obtained from *www.mitobi.com*.

OPC is the name of a product that combines ABM mushrooms with oleander, pau d'arco and cat's claw. All three herbs have strong anti-cancer credentials (though great care needs to be taken in the preparation of oleander as it is normally poisonous). OPC was patented in South Africa and has, apparently, been used there with great success. It is available at: *www.takesun.com*. (A cheaper source for this product is Marc Swanepoel, who owns the patent. See *www.sutherlandiaopc.com*.)

Note that although dramatic long-term effects have been seen with OPC, there may be some short-term side effects. Marc Swanepoel gives the following list: slight nausea and vomiting, diarrhoea, pruritus, pain at a tumour site, tachycardia and arrhythmia. Because of its blood-thinning properties, people on medical blood-thinning preparations should consult their doctors before using the OPC. People on heart-active drugs, such as digoxin (Lanoxin) or anti-arrhythmics, should also speak to their doctors before using the mixture. No other drug interactions have been reported. Pregnant women should not use the mixture. Other short-term detoxification symptoms like a slight rash, runny nose, pimples, slightly painful joints, etc., may be experienced. Marc also recommends a diet that is 70% fruit and 30% vegetable (preferably raw, otherwise steamed) – no meat or grains.

Recent research conducted at MD Anderson Cancer Centre has shown that oleander attacks cancer in a number of different ways: it inhibits angiogenesis, promotes apoptosis, stimulates the immune system, reduces the power of cancer cells to defend themselves, and promotes autophagy – a process where cells consume themselves. So, all in all, a very powerful aid.

Aloe vera

Aloe vera has demonstrated a strong ability to enhance the immune system's response to cancer. In addition it eliminates toxic wastes, which has a revitalizing effect on the body. It is also important for immune system defence. Most products make use of the inner gel, which is heat processed. This destroys many of the benefits. Look out for a whole-leaf, cold-pressed aloe vera product.

Essiac

In 1995, at the age of 28, Glynn Williams was diagnosed with Hodgkin's type lymphoma. 'I went to see the doctor because of swelling on both sides of the groin area which came on within about a week ... I was totally exhausted, lethargic, did not have the energy to get up, had no appetite, was losing weight and I was having chills.'

He started taking Essiac tea (brand name Flor-Essence) — two ounces in the morning before eating and two ounces at night. For a while the swelling continued to grow larger but then it hardened up and the discomfort went away. By this time test results confirmed that he had advanced stage Hodgkin's. He was put on a course of 16 chemotherapy treatments but after experiencing severe side effects he quit after the fifth session. Throughout this treatment he had continued with the Essiac tea (which he supplemented with vitamins and herbs, including black walnut tinctures, and wormwood capsules). He drank kombucha mushroom tea three times a day and did yoga with a strong focus on diaphragm breathing.

His doctors were amazed when he was eventually found to be cancer-free, as five doses of chemo was not considered curative. In December 2005, he confirmed that he was still cancer free.

Glynn was doing so many things that it is hard to isolate one and say that this cured him of cancer. However, the mainstay of his regime was Essiac tea and it comes with many testimonials as an effective cancer therapy.

The story is that a French Canadian nurse, René Caisse, was given an ancient Ojibway Indian healing formula. Whatever the truth of the story, she became famous for healing cancer using her herbal combination of burdock root, Turkish rhubarb, slippery elm and sheep sorrel. Nowadays these can be bought under a number of names: Tree of Life, Flor-Essence and Essiac itself. The name Essiac, incidentally, is simply Caisse reversed – a simple but effective way of branding the invention.

How it works is not known. Three of the four herbs used are considered foods and medicines, which are high in nutritive value. Sorrel has been used in Europe for centuries to help break down tumours. Burdock is a powerful blood purifier. Slippery elm is used traditionally as a tonic (helps strengthen the body) and seems to assist in healing. Rhubarb has a gentle laxative action which helps stimulate bile and also the gall bladder to expel toxic waste matter.

Very likely it works in a number of different ways. Perhaps there is a synergy between the parts so that when all four herbs are together in certain amounts they have an effect greater than any single herb would.

Melatonin

Melatonin is a hormone secreted by the pineal gland. It is in charge of our cycle of wakefulness and sleep. It is also an important regulator of our immune system. Interestingly, when we go to sleep so too does the cancer tumour. It stops growing, only switching on again the next day. Unfortunately our melatonin secretion drops as we grow older and we tend to sleep less well as a result. One suggestion is that melatonin should be taken as a supplement last thing at night. It may help to dissolve the melatonin in an oil base, such as coconut oil.

MGN-3

MGN-3 (also known as BioBran) is a potent immune system booster and helps to lessen the toxic side effects of conventional cancer treatment. It is made from the outer shell of rice bran which has been enzymatically treated with extracts from three different medicinal mushrooms: shiitake, kawaratake and suehirotake. One anecdotal report tells that MGN-3 was associated with the first recorded cure of multiple myeloma. In 1990, a 58-year-old man diagnosed with multiple myeloma who had had chemotherapy – which in any case is not expected to be curative – suffered a relapse. He started taking MGN-3 and within six months he was cancer-free and, when last recorded, was still alive and cancer-free eight years later. To what extent MGN-3 is curative of this or other cancers has not been determined. All that is claimed is that MGN-3 promotes the activity of natural killer cells.

It is now only available under the BioBran label. To be effective a daily dose of 2–3 grams needs to be taken for a month and 1 gram thereafter. It is widely available on the internet. For more information go to *www.biobran.org.*

Naltrexone (low dose naltrexone therapy)

Naltrexone is an FDA approved drug originally designed to help heroin addicts and alcoholics to quit (by making them ill if they persisted). However, in 1985, Bernard Bihari, MD, a New York City doctor, discovered that very low doses of this drug had a very powerful stimulating effect on the immune system. In addition to stabilizing AIDS, he found that this treatment also had a powerful, beneficial impact on many cancers including neuroblastoma, multiple myeloma and pancreatic cancer, which are normally considered incurable.

Interestingly, this treatment has the effect not of curing cancer but in many cases, where all other treatments have failed, of stopping it in its tracks. But please note that it is not 100% guaranteed to work. None of the approaches in this book carry such a claim. However, it is worth trying to see if you are one of the fortunate ones. But if it does work you will need to keep taking it permanently, otherwise the cancer could start growing again. So, this is not a stand-alone therapy. If you are lucky, it will buy you time in which you can experiment with other truly curative therapies.

LDN is safe, cheap and has no side effects (apart from possible sleeplessness in the first week or two of starting). While at normal doses naltrexone does interact very negatively with alcohol and opiate drugs, causing extreme nausea (which is why, under the name Antabuse, it has been used to wean alcoholics and drug addicts off their favoured substances of abuse), I am assured that at a low dose it is perfectly possible to enjoy a glass or two of wine. The standard dose of naltrexone is 50 mg but for our purposes we need only 2–4 mg taken once a day at bedtime. The easiest and cheapest way of doing this is to pulverize a 50 mg pill in a mortar and then dissolve it in 50 ml of distilled water. Then, using a dropper, you can extract the exact amount you need (1 mg = 1 ml of liquid). For further details go to *www.lowdosenaltrexone.org*.

Sunlight and sea water (vitamin D and minerals)

The importance of vitamin D was for a long time neglected – it was assumed that food sources were adequate. Little attention was paid to the fact that warnings against over-exposure to the sun were leading to a state where more and more children were being diagnosed with rickets. Now the 'don't go out in the sun' message has been successfully transmitted, we need to modify it by urging people to go out and get a healthy dose of sunlight.

Soaking up the sun's rays is a powerful means of strengthening the body's immune system. How long you should be out in the sun will obviously vary from place to place. You will not want to stay out in the searing heat of an Australian summer for as long as say a winter's day in England. In fact a winter's day in England is not going to do very much for you in terms of vitamin D acquisition. So if it's not warm enough to strip off and stretch out in the warmth of the sun, you should consider taking vitamin D tablets. Some of you may say that you get all your vitamin D from fish oils. If you do, then you will be eating a lot of fish oil. A tablespoon of cod liver oil will give you a little over 1000 iu of vitamin D. If you listen to most establishment sources of information, this is certainly enough. However, there are other vitamin D researchers who claim that food sources will always be inadequate in providing an optimal level of vitamin D intake. They note for example that exposing the whole body to warm sun for 15–20 minutes will give the body around 25,000 iu of vitamin D (equivalent to 25 tablespoons of cod liver oil). And how does the body feel after this amount of time? It feels great. There is in fact no known level of intake that creates vitamin D toxicity. Many people spend all day out in the sun and it doesn't make them nauseous. These same researchers are saying that oral supplementation of anywhere between 4000 iu and 10,000 iu during the winter months is a good way of maintaining the immune system. (Interestingly, people with black skin need to stay out longer in the sun to get the same benefit as people with lighter skins.)

When sunbathing, care should be taken to ensure the skin is not burnt. It is known that green tea is very protective of skin health, and a pot of cold green tea could be kept at hand to pour over you. Also, lavender oil and aloe vera gel are strong healers of sun-damaged skin. One could mix these ingredients together to make a home-made skin protection gel. Otherwise there are a number of organic sunscreens on the market. Of course, sunscreens (natural or otherwise) block the UV light you want to absorb, so make sure that the skin is naked to the sun for sufficient time to get the vitamin D benefits – between 20 minutes in a hot sun to an hour or more on a warm day. In very hot countries avoid the midday sun, but in less hot countries the midday sun will be precisely the best time of day for sunbathing. Obviously in winter in the cooler latitudes getting enough exposure to sunlight is going to be impossible, in which case a holiday may be in order. Please note that artificial sun beds or tanning booths are not recommended as alternatives.

While out in the bright sunlight, take off your glasses. The light is necessary for the stimulation of the pineal and other glands.

Having said all this, I take note of the fact that many official bodies with impeccable medical credentials strongly advise against too much exposure to the sun. The problem is that damage from the sun does have the potential to increase your likelihood of getting skin cancer. That said, however, we should also note that the types of skin cancer most often associated with over-exposure to the sun's rays are not normally fatal conditions. We should also note that this increased susceptibility in relation to skin cancers is counterbalanced by a far greater reduction in all other types of cancer – even deep-seated ones. This has been established by epidemiological studies of US Navy personnel who are often forced to spend long hours working in the hot sun. Yes, they do have a higher incidence of skin cancer. Against that, they have much lower levels of every other kind of cancer. These same establishment bodies also recommend shielding the eyes with sunglasses – to avoid cataracts. Yes, this is one of the decisions one has to make. Which would you rather have: cataracts or cancer?

Now let's turn our attention to swimming in the sea. The main benefit of being in the sea is that the body is able to absorb a perfect mix of mineral salts through the skin – especially magnesium. As we shall see in the next chapter, these minerals are potentially curative in their own right. For those who live at a distance from the sea, it is possible to purchase Himalayan or Dead Sea salt. These salt crystals can be dissolved in a warm bath and absorbed in that way.

Dandelion roots

Pick fresh dandelion roots (at any time of the year), cut off the leaves but don't wash off the soil. Put in an incubator and heat to 100°F for 5–6 days. (Alternatively dry in the sun or under a light bulb.) When it can be crumbled in the fingers, reduce to a fine powder in a pestle and mortar. Take half a teaspoon a day dissolved in water. This, according to American farmer George Cairns, is the secret to recovery from cancer. He was so convinced that this was the cure of his own cancer that he bought an advert in a Chicago newspaper to let the world know. The soil, he says, is good for you too.

Epicor

This is a substance that was originally used to produce fermented feed products for animals. However, alert managers at the feed processing plant noted that those who worked with the substance never seemed to fall ill. Research showed that these workers had very strong immune systems. This substance has now been packaged for human use. It is widely and cheaply available via the internet.

These then are some of the many ways in which the immune system can be boosted – and a strong immune system will help you live longer and feel better.

Bob Davis

In April 1996 Bob Davis discovered he had a massive cancer tumour – a foot wide and several inches thick – in his abdomen, and several other tumours in his chest, some 'the size of soft balls'. The cancer had also spread to his bone marrow.

He was immediately started on a very heavy chemotherapy programme to last three months. This had very little effect: 'It [the tumour] seemed to thrive on the stuff.' Eventually, his doctor told him that the chemo wasn't working. 'He later told me that another treatment would kill me. I knew that this was true because my body was ravaged by the chemo. I was curled up in a fetal position unable to sleep or eat. I was emaciated and had excruciating pain all through my body.'

At this time he received a call from a woman who had been selling his wife pills made of dried green barley leaves for her arthritis. During the conversation he mentioned his fight with cancer. 'Don't you know that cancer and arthritis can't grow in an alkaline body?' she said. The same barley leaves that his wife was taking for her arthritis would, she told him, also help him in his fight against cancer. He started taking the pills – 20 tablets of dried barley green (340 mg each) – and 'in ten days my cancer was 95% gone!' A number of tests including a CAT scan showed that scar tissue remained but the cancer had been killed. 'I was incredibly lucky. I know most people wouldn't be cured so simply. In fact I only know one other person who had the same response.'

A few years later, even though he had maintained his intake of dried barley leaves, Bob was diagnosed with a probable prostate cancer on the basis of a lump and high PSA levels. Resisting pressure to have surgery, Bob went on Dr Schulze's Incurable's programme which involved juice fasting and colon cleansing. Three weeks later he demanded a PSA re-test. His PSA levels were now normal.

In 2006 he was still cancer-free. He still takes 20 tablets of dried green barley every day. 'It costs me a whopping 95 cents or so.' He has adopted a 95% vegan diet. 'I really like it. I feel better than I have in 40 years. People say I look younger. I have lotsa energy.'

Bob Davis can be contacted through his website at *www.cancer-success.com*.

Feed the Body with the Right Nutrients

When we think of disease, we tend automatically to think in terms of the disease being caused by an agent: a virus or bacterium. But some diseases are known as deficiency diseases: they are the result of something lacking in the diet. Scurvy is the best known example, the result of too little vitamin C. Beriberi is another deficiency disease that decimated the population of Indonesia for several centuries before it was finally realized that the local diet was lacking in thiamine, vitamin B_1, the result of people rejecting red rice and instead eating mainly polished white rice. So this leads us to an interesting question: Is it possible that cancer could be a deficiency disease? If so, it could be cured simply by providing the missing nutrient.

In fact a number of people have made the suggestion that the root cause of cancer is the absence of a key nutrient. If so, which key nutrient is absent?

Folic acid

There are a number of candidates. The first I will consider is folic acid. This is the vitamin B_9. It is recognized that many if not most people are deficient in this vitamin, which is present in green leafy vegetables and, more and more commonly, in 'fortified' breakfast cereals. The drinking of orange juice or any other fruit juice containing vitamin C enhances absorption of folic acid from food. Many people are taking folic acid supplements of up to 1000 mcg. Alcohol and drugs can have a negative impact on our folic acid intake.

Folic acid is necessary for healthy cell division and to repair damage to DNA. It is known that most cervical dysplasias and other pre-cancerous conditions leading up to full blown cervical cancer will correct themselves once adequate folic acid intake is established. Many other cancers have been associated with low levels of folic acid. A good level of folic acid intake is known to be of value in treating many different forms of cancer. However, it is also difficult to get enough folic acid in your diet from vegetables alone. Actually liver is the food with the highest folic acid content, but supplementation is still advisable.

Vitamin C

Another candidate is vitamin C. It has been suggested that a deficiency of vitamin C is a possible cause of cancer. Many people think of it as simply an antioxidant. In fact vitamin C is one of the fundamental elements for our physical biochemistry. It is vital for a vast range of biochemical and enzymatic reactions, not to mention its role in maintaining the collagen that holds everything together. Scurvy is the result of things not holding together. Interestingly, some of the symptoms of leukaemia are identical to scurvy and I know of one anecdote in which a young child with leukaemia was cured after taking in large doses of vitamin C.

We have already discussed the potential for vitamin C to be curative. And there are a growing number of people who swear that intravenous vitamin C, three times a week for a number of weeks, has cured them of cancer. To restate the vitamin C argument, the main reason for supplementing with the vitamin is that most animals make vitamin C, and they make it in very large quantities. When they are ill they make it in even larger quantities. To extrapolate these results in human terms, given our size and weight the levels of vitamin C we would probably be producing if we could produce it range from 8–12 grams on a good day to 100 grams on a bad one. There must be a reason why these animals are producing so much vitamin C. If we are not producing or taking in anything like this level then we must be deficient. Therefore when we are ill it makes sense for us to take it in as large a quantity as we can, and in the form of L-ascorbic acid, which is mildly acidic, or in the form of sodium ascorbate (but not calcium ascorbate), which is not acidic at all.

Trace minerals

We have looked at folic acid and vitamin C. Let us now look at a third suggestion proposed by a New Zealand farmer,

Percy Weston, who was diagnosed with terminal cancer when he was 39 but who went on to die at the grand old age of 100. Before he was himself diagnosed with cancer, he had discovered his sheep were falling ill. 'We had a plague of cancer lesions coming up on the ears of the sheep,' he wrote. When he discovered their lesions, he analysed the situation and decided to test his theory that it was the superphosphate fertilizer that was to blame. He and other farmers had begun to use superphosphate fertilizers on their farms a few years previously. The initial result of using these fertilizers had been improved yields, but gradually the mineral content of the soil had become seriously degraded. To test this theory, he put his animals onto fresh pastures that had not been fertilized and provided them with natural rock phosphate and salt containing the missing minerals. The result? His sheep were healed. He repeated this test several times. When he put the animals on pastures fertilized with the superphosphates, they developed cancer. When they were moved to clean, organic pastures they recovered.

So, when he himself was diagnosed with cancer, he decided to mix together a mineral formula based on his experiences with his sheep. His cancer left him, and so did his arthritis. And he was still farming at the age of 97! He was free of cancer, arthritis and heart disease to the end. He wrote an extremely important book, *Cancer: Cause and Cure*, which details his clear demonstration that the main cause of cancer is the way we grow our food.

He discovered that the highly acidic chemical fertilizer superphosphate in addition to depleting the soil of minerals also killed the soil bacteria and earthworms necessary for the healthy regeneration of the soil. The result was – and remains – that the majority of our food contains excessive phosphorus and is deficient in calcium, magnesium, selenium, zinc, cobalt and other trace minerals.

It was fortunate for Percy Weston that his animals came down with cancer a year or so before he did.

An inexpensive multi-mineral mix, based on his ideas, is available under the name CAA capsules from the following website: *www.zealandpublishing.co.nz*. One of the key trace minerals in the mix is selenium. It is well known that cancer incidence is greater in areas with low selenium levels in the soil. High selenium intake is associated with reduced cancer risk. This is additional support for the idea that trace mineral deficiency could be a cause of cancer.

All of this leads strongly to the conclusion that the quality of the food we eat – and consequently the quality of our health – is very dependent on the quality of the soil our food grows in. For this reason organic food should be a standard part of our diet, and we need to be very protective about what food companies can call 'organic'.

There are other products that contain a rich mix of trace minerals and are also associated with cancer cures. One of these is Beres Drops. Formulated by a Hungarian scientist, Dr Jozsef Beres, Beres Drops is a liquid formula containing a patented combination of the following ingredients: distilled water, glycerol, EDTA, glycogen, iron, L-tartaric acid, zinc, sodium, succinic acid, magnesium, manganese, L-ascorbic acid, potassium, copper, molybdenum, vanadium, nickel, boron, fluorine, chlorine and cobalt. The concept behind the drops is that healthy cellular functioning requires these minerals in very specific combinations and dose levels. On 15 September 1991, the *Sun* newspaper carried the story of a Mrs Wendy Cook who claimed that three months on the drops had had the effect of shrinking a malignant tumour in her groin from 4 inches to one inch. She intended to continue with the drops rather than proceed with surgery.

Beres tested his drops on 235 cancer patients in Hungary and one third responded. So, useful though it undoubtedly is, it does not amount to a 100% certain cancer cure.

There is wide agreement that Beres Drops Plus is at the very least an important immune system support, not just for cancer but also AIDS and chronic fatigue among others. It should be noted that this is one of the very few products that contains vanadium, which is known to have strong anti-cancer effects of its own. It is also possible to get pure vanadium supplements. This essential trace mineral has no known toxic effects, even at quite large doses when taken orally. A source of ionic vanadium is *www.rainbowminerals.net*. Beres Drops are widely available from internet suppliers.

Another product, Oxy E, combines trace minerals in a solution designed to deliver oxygen into the cells efficiently, so combining two anti-cancer strategies. Interestingly the trace minerals are the means by which the oxygen gets into the cell, which explains why they are so important.

To return to Percy Weston, there is no doubt that he cured himself, his wife and many neighbours of cancer – his book contains many strong testimonials of the curative value of his mineral mix. But that does not necessarily mean that the same mineral mix will cure the cancer of someone living outside New Zealand, where cancers may be caused by other factors. The truth is cancer may have multiple causes. However, having said that, a multi-mineral mix, along with a good size dose of folic acid and vitamin C might very well be exactly what the doctor ordered – if he was so minded to. But sadly these are not patentable medicines, so it is unlikely that he will be so minded.

We have now dealt with the strategies aimed at returning the body to a state of health. In the next five chapters I will look at five distinct approaches that focus directly on the cancer tumour itself.

Shirley Lipschutz-Robinson

In 1982, doctors recommended a mastectomy on Shirley's left breast. She had suffered recurring cyst lumps which no medication could control. Up until this time Shirley was, as she calls herself, a prescription drug junkie. She was depressed, overweight and suffering from a seemingly endless parade of ailments, and the drugs seemed only to make matters worse. Her overall health was steadily declining.

But Shirley baulked at having her breast removed. She decided she needed to change her approach. She consulted a naturopathic/homoeopathic doctor who put her on a dietary regime, 'a wholesome diet of fresh, organically grown fruits, vegetables, and nuts, mostly in their raw form', supplemented with homoeopathic remedies. The results were, in her own words, 'dramatic'.

Within six weeks the lumps were gone. Within twelve weeks she had lost 60 lb. 'My energy level and stamina improved dramatically. I was able to function better overall. I became calmer, centred and focused, and generally I felt happier. My overall resistance to infections became excellent.'

In the 1990s, she experienced a lump the size of a pea in her left nipple. It grew to be the size of a small grape. She refused to see the doctor, instead self-treating it with extra flaxseed oil, herbal extracts and homoeopathy. Within two weeks her body had reabsorbed the lump and it never came back.

These experiences sparked her to study a wide range of alternative therapies. Her full story, and the story of how she treated her husband through a series of heart attacks, is told on her excellent website: *www.shirleys-wellness-cafe.com*. This website is a storehouse of useful information.

Cut the Cancer's Energy Supply

If you take all the petrol out of a car it isn't going to go very far. It's the same with a cancer cell. Cut the fuel lines and it will stop dead in its tracks.

We have already learnt that the key difference between a cancer cell and a normal healthy one is the means by which it gets its energy. Normal cells get their energy through an oxidative process while cancer cells use a fermentation process that involves glycolysis. Glycolysis is the name given to the metabolic pathway that uses sugar as a fuel and converts it under conditions of low oxygenation – anaerobic respiration – into ATP (adenosine triphosphate), which in turn is the key biochemical component that allows cells to keep running. It is necessary both for intracellular energy transfer and also for DNA replication.

ATP depletion therapy is an approach that is getting serious attention from mainstream researchers. But we don't need to wait for results that can be turned into a patented medicine. We already have ways that make use of this approach to attack cancer.

The first energy-depletion strategy is so simple that you should kick yourself for not seeing it already: cut sugar out of your diet completely. This doesn't mean that you should switch to 'sugar-free' products that use artificial sweeteners such as aspartame (which research is showing to be highly toxic) or saccharine. The only sugars to be excluded from the not-to-be-consumed list are the fruit sugars in their original wrapping. You can eat apples, grapes, oranges, etc. The fructose in these products is less bio-available than glucose or sucrose. Also these fruits are powerhouses of other healthy phytonutrients (a fancy word for plant-based nutrients) which can help fight the cancer. So sugar is out while raw organic fresh fruit is in. Those of you who have an incurably sweet tooth should consider using Stevia, a herbal sweetener that is also healthy.

Secondly, to further our fuel-depletion strategy, we can interfere with the glycolytic process itself by drinking diluted apple cider vinegar. A splash of vinegar in a glass of water is all you need. Orange and lemon juice has a similar effect.

Then there is the ATP itself. One group of Indian researchers have formulated the thesis that one way of attacking cancer is to inhibit ATP with a substance called methylglyoxal.

Methylglyoxal

This is itself a natural breakdown product that we produce in our bodies during glycolysis. In 2001, Indian biochemist

Professor Manju Ray trialled methylglyoxal on 19 patients with 'very advanced stages' of cancer. Of these, all of whom would normally have died within months, only three did in fact die; five had their cancers stabilized and eleven were effectively cured. Further studies resulted in an overall cure rate of 70% in cancer patients who were diagnosed as terminally ill. It is very likely the cure rate would have been higher if taken at earlier stages.

Even better, methylglyoxal, unlike other chemotherapy drugs, is virtually non-toxic for normal cells. Methylglyoxal has every appearance therefore of being a safe and highly effective treatment for cancer. In short, all those women who sold their houses in order to afford Herceptin should really have been trying to get their hands on methylglyoxal. So, can we all go home and relax? Sadly not. When in 2006 I asked Cancer Research UK what research was being done on methylglyoxal and cancer I was informed that to all extents and purposes there was no such research being done in the UK. The information officer at Cancer Research UK even disputed the very well publicized fact that human trials in India had been very successful. Having shown him where he could find the information, I expected further discussion. In fact I did not hear from him again.

However, this story is not quite a cul de sac. We do have a source of methylglyoxal at our disposal. What's more, it is free of charge and very conveniently available. Where? In your urine. In fact urine has been touted for many centuries, perhaps millennia, as a health tonic equal to any, and better than most. Besides methylglyoxal, it contains large amounts of urea and indeed it is a rich cocktail of organic substances. Many millions of people regularly drink a glassful and swear to its beneficial effects. I once talked to a medical missionary in Mexico who was working with impoverished peasants who had cancer. She was getting good results simply by putting them on a vegetarian diet and getting them to drink their own urine.

The very idea of drinking urine is repugnant to many people, yet it is well known that it is a clean substance and that it even has antibiotic properties. You can, for example, put urine on a cut to help prevent infection. In order to make urine more palatable it is advisable to go vegetarian, as this makes the taste less objectionable. You can mix it with (freshly squeezed) orange juice or supergreen powders to mask the taste. The best urine comes from the middle urine of the first urination of the morning, but in truth any urine will do. Some holistic and ayurvedic therapists such as the Australian Walter Last recommend a urine fast in which, for three or four weeks, nothing is taken in except the person's own urine.

Another strategy that is being looked at with great interest, by both mainstream and alternative researchers, is to attack cancer by interfering with the development of its blood supply. In order for tumours to grow bigger they induce the adult body to grow a blood supply, a process known as angiogenesis. The search is on, therefore, for anti-angiogensis weapons that will stop the development of blood vessels. The notorious drug thalidomide is being given a new lease of life as just such an anti-angiogenesis agent.

Cancer is one of three instances where the body will produce new blood vessels. The other two are: the inflammation that is the result of injury (or other cause); and pregnancy and the development of the foetus. Clearly anything that interferes with the blood supply of a cancer tumour will also interfere with the healthy continuation of pregnancy. If you are pregnant please take note.

What anti-angiogenesis agents are there that we can make use of?

For many years shark cartilage was touted as the great answer to cancer precisely because – as its main proponents argued – sharks don't get cancer. Sadly, however, some sharks apparently do get cancer. Shark cartilage remains available, along with bovine cartilage, but is very expensive in the quantities required for our purpose. Much more readily available are miso soup, the mineral selenium and the North American herb bindweed. But perhaps the most effective of all these readily available anti-angiogenesis factors is curcumin.

Curcumin is an extract from the herb turmeric and it is getting very serious attention from cancer researchers. It should be mentioned here that curcumin is now known to attack cancer in other ways – not just through its inhibition of angiogensis – and we will discuss under Strategy 12 another of its important effects.

For the cancer patient pure curcumin is required and a dose of 4–8 grams a day is recommended. However, curcumin capsules are useless as the curcumin needs to be dissolved in fat before being ingested. The best way to take it is to buy curcumin powder and dissolve it in warm coconut milk or cream and drink it. According to one testimony I have seen it has a very powerful effect. However, a word of caution: it should not be used in the case of any brain cancer as it may cause the cancer to swell. Curcumin works synergistically with feverfew herb, which is also not soluble in water so it too needs to be dissolved in fat (effective dose around 4 grams per day).

And finally, as we have seen, vitamin D from sunlight also works against cancer in a number of ways – one of them is by inhibiting angiogenesis. One scientist, Steve Martin, believes that vitamin D (5000 iu) mixed with melatonin (6 mg) powdered and dissolved in warm coconut milk (which itself is loaded with lauric acid, a healthy fat even if it is a 'saturated fat') and taken at night on an empty stomach is as good a cancer preventative as any, and that higher doses might even be curative. Steve Martin posts an interesting science blog at *www.grouppekurosawa.com*.

June Black

June Black was first diagnosed with cancer (stage 1) in November 2000. She eventually had a mastectomy but no radiation or chemotherapy. She was put on tamoxifen but reacted badly to it and 'threw it down the toilet'. In 2005, June noticed a lump growing on the mastectomy scar and had it biopsied. The tests came back positive. The cancer had returned. She underwent two further operations but it was clear the cancer had spread. By this time she had read a lot of books and had come round to the natural approach to treating cancer. So when her third oncologist (she had dumped two) told her, 'I recommend the whole gamut; chemo, radiation and adjuvant hormone therapy,' she found the courage to refuse, saying: 'I am 60 years old, I have lived a good life, and I have other plans.'

But at first the natural path did not appear to be doing her any good. 'After spending a month on a very strict diet and enough vitamins and supplements to fill a small shop I realized I was losing the war against this cancer. I was losing weight, I had sweats, I was really weak and it was so bad that I thought death would be a wonderful alternative to the hell I was going through.'

Then someone suggested the supplement PolyMVA. She went on it and within four days felt better. This was in October 2005. In June 2006 she had a full array of tests and they all came back clear. She was cancer free.

Her regime was eight teaspoons of PolyMVA a day for six and a half months. She then went to six teaspoons a day for about two months and since then has been taking four teaspoons a day. She also takes COQ10, artemisinin, pancreatic enzymes and IP_6.

'This is just the tip of the iceberg of what I am taking. I also take different mushrooms, Epicor, Lugol's Iodine, DIM, Calcium-d-Glucarate. If anyone is interested in my complete list please feel free to contact me at *june1@mesquiteweb.com*. I just had my 62nd birthday, March 1, 2007, in Hawaii and gained more weight and feel fantastic. As of now, no signs of illness. I have excellent health and work full time and care for 11 cats.'

June's story is one of many testimonials that can be found at *www.polymvasurvivors.com*.

Interfere with the Cancer Cell's DNA

One of the attributes that distinguishes the cancer cell from most normal cells is the rate of cell division. Cancer cells divide more often in the same time frame than do most — but not all — normal cells. One way of attacking cancer therefore is to interfere with its ability to divide.

One approach focuses on an enzyme called nuclear factor-kappa B (NF-κB). When this enzyme is present in increased quantities then cell division is encouraged. If a way can be found to inhibit this enzyme then cell division will be reduced or even blocked entirely.

In fact there are a number of natural substances that can achieve this objective. We have, in fact, met most of them before. The usual suspects in this case include vitamin C, vitamin D (yes, more sunbathing!), curcumin and one or two other substances.

For vitamin C to be effective in this way it needs to be present at very high intracellular levels. This means taking it intravenously, as we have already discussed, or in the form of Lypo-Spheric vitamin C (obtainable from *www.livonlabs.com*).

Ellagic acid is a naturally occurring polyphenolic con-stituent found in many different fruits and nuts, in red raspberries in particular but also in strawberries, blueberries and walnuts. It is also, it seems, a highly potent anti-carcinogen which has the ability to inhibit mutations within a cell's DNA. In some studies cancer activity was stopped within 48 hours.

There is a lot of excitement about the potential benefits of this chemical and even the American Cancer Society has not been able to ignore it — though it unhelpfully informed readers that it is not available as a supplement. Technically they were correct — any supplement claiming to contain ellagic acid is a fraud. However, supplements containing ellagitannins will provide the raw materials which are converted to ellagic acid in the body. The raspberry's seeds contain the highest concentrations of ellagitannin.

I would start my internet search at *www.ellagic.net* and compare this product with others available from other sources. For skin cancer there is Raspex SPF-30 skin gel which is made from Meeker raspberries and has a strong ellagitannin content. See *www.smdi.org*.

Skin cancers

Non-fatal skin cancers pose a very specific problem and people diagnosed with these types of cancer should consider the following treatments.

Curaderm (BEC5)

This is a cream which has demonstrated strong healing activity against a number of skin cancers. It was developed by Dr Bill Cham, an Australian biochemist and is based on a plant, *Solanum sodomaeum*, which is known in Australia as devil's apple or kangaroo apple. It is not a burning salve like bloodroot but its effectiveness has been demonstrated in a number of studies at reputable London hospitals. The cream is also promoted as beneficial for psoriasis and eczema.

BEC5 can eradicate non-melanoma skin cancers, specifically basal cell carcinomas (BCC) and squamous cell carcinomas (SCC). It is also effective against benign tumours and other skin irregularities, such as keratoses, sun spots and age spots.

One important point to note is that it is vital to use the cream before any surgery has taken place. This is because cancerous tissues on the skin are connected to cancerous tissues below the surface. The cream can then eliminate all these cancerous cells one after the other. Surgery may eliminate surface cells without impacting on the cells below the surface. The cream then cannot get access to the deeper lying cells. (It is available from *www.curaderm.net* and a number of other websites.)

See also Raspex SPF-30 skin gel (*www.smdi.org*), and a person with skin cancer has also recommended PDQ Cream to me as being beneficial. Go to *www.behealed.biz* for further details.

Warning: If you have skin cancer, be very careful what the

oncologist recommends. One skin cancer medication, Aldara, which contains the chemical imiquimod (IQ) has been known since 1986 to be itself a cause of cancer. 'It is so dangerous that the American Cancer Society, the National Cancer Institute and others have determined it is a carcinogen, and have placed it on their lists of most hazardous chemicals. The US Occupational Safety Health Agency has even listed IQ as a laboratory chemical hazard. Yet, doctors worldwide are prescribing it, willy-nilly, to "cure" skin cancers...' (Elaine Hollingsworth, an Australian skin cancer patient who nearly died using it, writing in *The Townsend Newsletter*, May 2006 edition). See also her own website: *www.doctorsaredangerous.com*.

Finally, people with skin cancers can make a paste by adding a few drops of water to vitamin C powder and rubbing this on exposed cancerous areas several times a day, leaving it to dry on the skin. There are anecdotal reports that this has caused surface cancers to heal within a week or two.

Seanol

Another natural product that boasts interesting credentials is Seanol, the registered trade name for an extract of marine algae. In addition to being an antioxidant, it has shown marked benefits for circulatory problems from blood pressure and arthritis to sexual dysfunction. And it appears to slow down tumour cell division. It is sold under the trade names of Fibronol and Fibroboost.

Cranberries

Finally, recent research has shown that cranberries contain phytochemicals that interfere with cell division.

Bruce Guilmette

In November 2004, Bruce discovered that both his kidneys had large cancerous masses inside them. Kidney cancer is known to be highly resistant to treatment and he was given only a matter of months to live unless he had both kidneys removed. Bruce refused this option, and turned to a combination of diet, supplements and the use of a Rife machine. Bruce's research led him to the conclusion that cancer needs to be attacked from many different angles to be successfully put into remission. He eventually put together a complex regimen that he followed rigorously. Much of his food intake is in the form of juiced fresh vegetables. He reduced his meat consumption to no more than 10% of his total intake and eliminated pork altogether. He has come to accept that the dietary changes he made to defeat cancer will become a lifelong practice. Bruce died on 30 November 2007, but he did not die of cancer. All his blood tests indicated that the cancer was no longer active. His full story is told at *www.survivecancerfoundation.org.*

Induce Cancer Cell Suicide

As we learnt in the preamble to this book, cancer cells are normal cells that have been forced to change their means of getting energy. They have been forced to use an anaerobic pathway because of the relatively low oxygen levels of the surrounding tissues. In order to do this the cell has had to switch off the mitochondria, which in normal circumstances act as the cell's batteries. However, the mitochondria also have another function. They manage the process of apoptosis. Apoptosis is the formal term for what can also be called normal pre-programmed cell death. All normal cells die and are replaced by new cells that start life as generic stem cells but which become normalized by their context. A stem cell that finds itself in the brain becomes another brain cell. An otherwise identical stem cell that finds itself in the liver will become a liver cell. When their vitality is depleted they are programmed by their DNA to die and they are replaced. This is a dynamic process that is in continual play. The trouble with cancer cells is that they have lost this ability. If we can reverse the process and switch on the mitochondria, then the cell will rediscover its ability to die naturally and it will activate this process.

Fortunately this is not just theory. A large number of compounds do have this ability to normalize cancer cells and induce apoptosis. In this chapter we will look at some of these. And we have already met a number of these substances: curcumin powder, selenium, vanadium, vitamin D (yes, still more sunbathing) and ellagic acid. But let's turn our attention to others that we have not yet met.

IP_6

IP_6 is a chemical called inositol hexaphosphate and is found naturally in high fibre foods such as beans, brown rice and wheat bran. A number of animal studies, but as yet no human studies, indicate that it is extremely effective against a wide range of cancers. It appears to work against all cancer cells by normalizing them – turning them back into normal cells. Interestingly, it has been found to work against every kind of cancer cell studied in animals – and there is no known toxicity.

According to Dr Abdul Kalam Shamsuddin, Professor of Pathology at the University of Maryland School of Medicine in Baltimore, who developed IP_6, someone with cancer should be taking 4800–7200 mg of IP_6 and 1200–1800 mg of inositol. One reputable brand is Cell Forte. It is widely available on the internet. Dr Shamsuddin recommends two scoops in the morning and two in the evening.

Vitamin E succinate

Vitamin E is a substance viewed with some disfavour in relation to cancer. There are some suspicions that standard forms of vitamin E may actually protect cancer. However, there is one form of vitamin E, alpha-tocopherol succinate, which has been found to promote apoptosis. A good source for this vitamin is Life Extension Foundation at *www.lef.org*.

Cayenne pepper

Cayenne pepper is known to be very effective for heart problems and can even stop a heart attack. Herbalist Dr Richard Schulze also claims that it has powerful anti-cancer effects. He tells the story of a man who had an inoperable brain tumour. He went home, did a colon/liver detox, and then started a regime of ten cups per day of cayenne pepper tea. In three months he returned to his doctor and his X-rays showed a dried up, dead tumour in his head.

In March 2006, the journal *Cancer Research* published the results of a study undertaken at Los Angeles' Cedars-Sinai Medical Centre demonstrating that capsaicin, the ingredient that makes peppers hot, has the effect of causing cancer cells to die by inducing apoptosis (programmed cell death).

Schulze recommends one teaspoon of organic cayenne pepper, or an equivalent number of drops of a good cayenne pepper tincture, in a glass of hot water three times a day for almost everything. If you are not used to hot foods, you will have to build up very slowly to this level. Start with even as little as one sixteenth of a teaspoon.

Capsules should be avoided as the interaction of the cayenne in the mouth is an important feature of its benefits.

Cayenne also has the immediate impact of widening the blood vessels, which allows more blood and oxygen to reach distant sites. This means that besides being effective in itself it will also speed the delivery of other drugs and herbs you take at the same time.

Digitalis

Digitalis, a well-known extract from foxglove used for certain heart conditions, has been found to have a very potent anti-cancer effect for a wide variety of cancers. It appears to work by inducing apoptosis. However, the extract is currently available in two forms — one of which has no anti-cancer effect. Digitoxin, from *Digitalis purpurea*, is effective; the similarly named and now more commonly used digoxin, from *Digitalis lanata*, has no anti-cancer effect.

In a Swedish study, breast cancer patients who were on digitalis had a 90% reduction in recurrence of cancer over five years compared with a control group. Twenty-two years later only 6% of the digitalis group had died from breast cancer compared with almost 50% of the control group. As Dr Wayne Martin has commented, 'Digitalis is the right drug being used to treat the wrong disease.'

DMSO

Dimethyl sulphoxide (DMSO) is an organic sulphur compound. It is a clear, colourless and largely odourless liquid that has demonstrated clear anti-tumour qualities. Over 6000 articles in the scientific literature establish a very solid claim to be recognized as an anti-cancer weapon. Vets use it freely when treating cancer in animals. It is available on the internet from *www.dmso.com* and *www.dmso.org* (two distinct companies).

DMSO can be taken by intravenous injection, orally, or it can be rubbed on. It is absorbed very rapidly through the skin, and this is a very efficient way of getting it to the intended site.

DMSO has a wide range of biological activities. One reason given for this is that it creates very powerful bonds with water molecules. This allows it to penetrate membranes and to pass from one organ or tissue to another with great ease. It has a wider range of biochemical actions than any other known chemical agent. Skin cancers respond quickly to treatment with DMSO, and it is also effective against brain tumours. It has been suggested that a good way of getting caesium chloride into the body is to dissolve it first in DMSO.

Are there any side effects to taking DMSO? A garlicky taste in the mouth and bad smell on the breath. Some people suffer from headaches, dizziness and mild nausea. A localized skin rash or burning feeling can occur on the skin.

Warning: DMSO is an extremely powerful solvent. It will dissolve anything, including latex gloves and plastic. Obviously no one wants anything poisonous to be dissolved and taken into the body, so all jewellery should be taken off and the skin's surface should be cleaned thoroughly before DMSO is used. DMSO should never come in contact with plastic – only glass and a high quality stainless steel spoon. A dose level of 1–2 teaspoons a day should be sufficient.

MSM supplements are made from DMSO and are thought to have many of DMSO's advantages without the negative smell or potential for toxicity. MSM appears to inhibit pain and improve blood flow. It is important for collagen (needed for cell walls) and helps the body maintain a good pH level. And there is evidence that it slows the growth of cancer tumours, and may even turn malignant tumours into benign tumours. Some people have combined DMSO and MSM to good effect. MSM is widely and cheaply available and is used as a treatment for arthritis.

Dichloroacetate (DCA)

In January 2007 an article in *New Scientist* magazine alerted the world to what may be a cheap, out of patent, cure for cancer. In lab tests conducted at the University of Alberta, the drug DCA, which has been used for many years to treat a number of rare metabolic disorders, was found to kill cancer cells in vitro and also in animal studies. DCA appears to reawaken the mitochondria, and this in turn switches on apoptosis – causing the cancer cells to die. The drug is taken orally in water and is fairly safe, though there are some uncomfortable side effects including pain or numbness. Whether or not it becomes widely available in the near future remains to be seen, but it may be worth mentioning it to your doctor.

Ginger tea

And if none of these appeals you could simply chop up some fresh ginger and let it steep for a while in boiling water. Drink the resulting ginger tea. Yes, this too will help persuade cancer cells to become normal.

Cimetidine

In 1979 *The Lancet* carried a letter from two doctors at Nebraska University describing the curious fact that two of their cancer patients had both had spontaneous remissions while taking the non-prescription drug cimetidine, also known as Tagamet, commonly used to treat gastric ulcers and other digestive disorders. One had squamous cell carcinoma and the other large cell lung cancer. In August 1982 three other doctors reported in *The Lancet* that a patient with stage 4 melanoma had started taking 1000 mg of cimetidine and had had an almost instantaneous recovery, with tumours disappearing within a few weeks (Thornes, R. D., Lynch, G., Sheehan, M. V., 'Cimetidine and coumarin therapy of melanoma', *Lancet* 1982; ii: 328). Over the years there have been many similar anecdotes with a wide range of cancers. Cimetidine is relatively safe though it does have the potential to interact with other drugs, and in males there is the possibility of breast enlargement. Against that it could be remarkably effective. Little research has been done on why it works.

Mark Olsztyn

In March 1991, Mark experienced a major epileptic seizure which led to him being hospitalized. There, a CAT scan revealed a darkened area in the right frontal lobe of his brain. He was operated on and the tumour removed. It was found to be a low-grade astrocytoma. No further treatment was recommended though frequent repeat scans would, he was told, be necessary.

Mark ignored this recommendation and for the next six years led a normal, hectic life. 'This was my denial phase,' he recalls. When eventually he did go for a scan, in 1997, he was shocked to learn that the tumour had returned and was now stage 4. In addition to surgery he would require chemotherapy and radiation. He was also told by one of his doctors that he had better settle his affairs. But Mark insisted in thinking positively that a cure was possible.

He followed doctor's orders and underwent all these treatments even though he knew that at best they would be palliative. Fortunately, his father was a doctor of alternative medicine. 'My father immediately sent me a case of a foul-tasting liquid called PolyMVA which a colleague of his was using successfully on brain tumour patients. Because PolyMVA can be used as an adjunct to conventional therapy I embraced it. I felt then that any nonconventional therapy that came my way, so long as it didn't interfere with what the doctors wanted me to do, was what God wanted me to do and would give me the edge that I needed to survive.

'Among many other things, I became an ascetic, practiced Qi Gong, drank Essiac and Chinese herbs, joined various support groups, received acupuncture, ohmed and prayed and was prayed for, drank shark cartilage, ate macrobiotic, practiced visualization and, after four out of six rounds, quit chemotherapy. That last one was not what the doctors wanted me to do, however I felt I had had enough poisoning.

'Over the years I gradually let go of each of the aforementioned life-saving practices except for PolyMVA and eating organic. Doctors now tell me to keep on doing whatever it is that I'm doing because it seems to be working.'

In January 2008, Mark was very much alive and cancer free.

Strategy 13:

Attack the Tumour

Already it will be evident that the rather cuddly distinction that is usually made between orthodox and alternative therapies — that one treats the symptoms while the other is holistically concerned with the whole body — is very far from being a good description of reality. In my view, the key distinction is this. The orthodox approach to cancer is a restricted regime of toxic and not very effective therapies around which a defensive laager has been built. To answer why that has happened would probably fill another book. The alternative label, on the other hand, can be applied to every other approach under the sun. It is alternative simply because it is neglected or, if not neglected, actively opposed by mainstream medicine.

This is an important point to make because, although direct targeting of the tumour is an approach which has generally been seen as the preserve of orthodox medicine, there are in fact a number of alternative approaches that have the ability to attack and kill cancer cells either directly or indirectly without seeking to enhance the health of the whole body. I describe some of these approaches below.

Artemisinin and iron

Cancer patients are normally advised not to take iron supplements and to reduce their intake of foods rich in iron (liver, meat, dates, molasses, pizzas, etc.). The reason for this is that iron is needed for cell division. Since cancer cells have an increased need for iron to support their greater rate of cell division, they have more iron receptors on their surface to help iron to enter the cell. Therefore, in normal circumstances – normal for a cancer patient, that is – it makes sense to reduce as far as possible one's iron intake.

However, researchers have noted that artemisinin, an extract of wormwood herb, which has shown itself to be useful in the fight against malaria, is highly reactive in the presence of iron, releasing a burst of free radicals that results in killing the cell. So, although it is normally not advisable to take iron supplements in the case of cancer, when taking artemisin the reverse is true, as we wish to flood the cancer cells with iron.

Obviously, if you decide to try this approach, you need to reduce your intake of antioxidants as these will neutralize the free radicals. While we normally hear of free radicals in the context of oxidative damage to cells (we take antioxidants to prevent this damage), this is a case of free radicals being the goodies not the baddies. So while you are pursuing the artemisinin-iron approach cut out vitamin C, ellagic acid and any other substance that has antioxidant activity.

Bloodroot

Bloodroot, *Sanguinaria canadensis*, is native to the woods of north-central United States and Canada. This herb has demonstrated very powerful anti-cancer properties, especially for those with melanoma or other surface tumours. Quite simply, it dissolves any form of malignant growth while leaving healthy tissue alone. An extraordinary set of photographs showing this effect can be seen at *www.silvermedicine.org* and also at *www.cancerx.org*.

Bloodroot is easily and quickly absorbed into the body. So it is possible that the bloodroot will seek out tumours and eliminate them, even though they are not on the surface. One patient I have talked to used it to get rid of breast tumours – and over the next month found cancerous material being expelled from her neck as well. It was, she reports, extremely painful but certainly not as painful as chemotherapy. By the end of the month she was cancer free.

A number of black salves are available via the internet. The best known are TumorX Salve and Cansema. However, the Cansema brand products are no longer available. The manufacturer, Alpha Omega Labs, was put out of business by the FDA and the proprietor, Greg Caton, imprisoned for supposedly running a 'cancer cure scam'. However, information about TumorX salve is available at *www.cancerX.org*. The product is available at *www.simpledefeat.com*. A bloodroot tincture for internal use is available from *www.cancersalves.com*. Another black salve is sold under the name Balm of Gilead at *www.austinpages.com.*

It is not entirely clear how or why these so-called escharotic black salves work. One suggestion has been that it is the zinc chloride rather than the herb that is the key ingredient. Whatever the case, these pastes have demonstrated a clear ability to kill tumour cells while leaving healthy skin tissue only mildly irritated.

CanCell

CanCell is a mix of chemicals selected, it would appear, on the basis of their electrical charge. In fact little is known about the ingredients, which have changed from time to time, or the means by which it achieves its objective of eliminating cancer. But, despite all this murky uncertainty, it does appear to have a strong anti-cancer effect. One estimate is that for every 100 people taking it, 55 will experience a cure. There are a number of CanCell-like products on the market, the best known being CanCell itself, Cantron and Protocel. Other names that have been used are Entelev, Sheridan's Formula, Jim's Juice and Crocinic Acid. Given that the formulas for these different products are different to a greater or lesser extent, it may be worth considering using one and then, if there is no beneficial reaction, using another formula.

For further information go to the CanCell information site at *www.alternativecancer.us/cancell.*

Digestive enzymes

A number of our digestive enzymes are produced by the pancreas. Unfortunately, cancer is an efficient producer of chemicals that destroy these enzymes. This forces the pancreas to work harder to produce more enzymes. The result can quickly be an exhausted pancreas, especially as the pancreas may have been weak in the first place.

To help the pancreas you should drink green juices, cut back on eating meat, occasionally fast, and supplement your diet with pancreatic enzymes. Pancreatic enzymes should be taken when your system is most alkaline, particularly about 2–3 p.m. in the afternoon.

There are a number of different kinds of proteolytic digestive enzyme: proteases digest proteins, lipases digest fats, and amylases help to digest carbohydrates.

Enzymes not only attack cancer cells directly but also promote immune activity by helping stimulate production of a substance called tumour necrosis factor (TNF) which attacks cancer cells. They also interfere with metastatic activity, so stopping the cancer cells from spreading.

Commercial enzyme formulations often combine pancreatin with papain, a powerful enzyme derived from the papaya, and bromelain, an enzyme derived from the pineapple.

The most highly rated enzyme product is made by the German Wobe Mugos company and is marketed as Wobenzyme. This is widely available. Another is Vitalzyme.

Pancreatic enzymes should play an important part in any overall anti-cancer strategy (except when taking CanCell or when following the Budwig protocol) and should be taken in large quantities.

Dr William Kelley, who formulated the Kelley approach to cancer (see *Cancer: The Complete Recovery Guide* for further details), recovered from his own terminal pancreatic cancer using digestive enzymes. Pancreatic cancer is generally considered to be 100% terminal in a very short time, so anyone recovering from this form of cancer has very likely discovered some great truth.

Fasting

When the body has no fuel – from food sources – to burn, then it is forced to turn on itself. First go the fat supplies that have been built up, but when that's gone what then? The body is forced to make decisions about which other bits of itself it should consume – the muscles? Perhaps. The theory is that it will consume the part of itself that is most expendable. And what could be more expendable than a cancer tumour? That at least is the theory and there are certainly stories that bear this out. Dr Solomon Bard, who for many years ran the medical clinic at Hong Kong University, told me of a case that he had personally witnessed in a Japanese internment camp during the occupation of Hong

Kong. He was at that time a medical student and knew that one of his fellow internees had testicular cancer which had returned having been treated unsuccessfully with radiation. This man had perhaps a few weeks or months to live. Dr Bard was therefore very surprised to bump into him at the end of the war, and again ten years later. He was completely free of cancer. The cure? Dr Bard said it could only have been the Japanese camp diet – a starvation-level regime of cabbage soup and some rice.

The danger with fasting is that once the fast is over the cancer will return again. However, it is a strategy that may buy time. For those concerned about the inevitable hunger pangs, there is an appetite suppressing herb, Hoodia, used by the Bushmen of the Kalahari Desert when their food supplies are low.

Grape diet

The grape diet is a diet that consists entirely of eating red grapes – organic where possible and containing seeds, which need to be crushed in the teeth. Some recommend the possible addition of a supergreen mix such as Barley Power or Barlean's Greens. Grapes should be thoroughly washed if not organic. Eat grapes for breakfast, lunch and dinner – and elevenses and teatime and as a late night snack. Maintain this regime for about four weeks. Since most grapes seem to be seedless these days, you might consider finding a separate source of grape seed extract.

The reason the grape diet works, according to those who favour it, is that the cancer greedily sucks in the grape sugars – which contain a potent arsenal of poisons: resveratrol and quercetin above all. It is these poisons that kill the cancer. You can find resveratrol, quercetin and grape seed extract as individual supplements, but the grape diet does work for a wide variety of ailments, not just cancer, so it is very likely that there are other health-maintaining processes at work.

On a personal note, I did try to do this diet once myself. I can warn you not to expect an active social life while you're on it. Your eliminations will smell rather powerfully. This is a very good sign of the grape's ability to detoxify the body.

Graviola (and pawpaw)

Graviola is a South American tree which seems to have a miraculous combination of effects: it is harmless to normal cells yet there are claims that it is many times more potent as a cancer killer than Adriamycin, a chemotherapy drug. Pawpaw (here I am referring to a North American tree, not the other name for the papaya) is a cousin of graviola and considered to be even stronger as a cancer killer. Interestingly, they both appear to be effective against cancer cells that have shown themselves to be resistant to radiation and chemotherapy.

Laetrile

Laetrile is the name given by one of its early promoters, Ernst Krebs, to a substance found in concentrated form in apricot kernels and bitter almonds. Also known as amygdalin, nitriloside and vitamin B_{17}, it is found in varying quantities in up to two and a half thousand other plants, the vast majority of which are edible. While laetrile is available on the internet, you can get sufficient for the purpose of treating cancer from natural food sources. Just do an internet search for 'bitter almonds'.

The results of animal studies indicate that laetrile needs to be taken with vitamin A and digestive enzymes (Wobe Mugos or Vitalzym for example) to be really effective.

How does laetrile work? There have been two theories. The first is that it is a vitamin and that its deficiency has led to the vitamin-deficiency disease of cancer. For that reason it is sometimes called Vitamin B_{17}. However, it is the second theory that carries most respectability.

According to this theory, laetrile is a parcel that contains poisons. When the parcel is unwrapped the poisons are released. Normal cells do not have the power to unwrap the parcel. Only cancer cells have that power. Laetrile is a sub-stance that can be separated (by certain enzymes, in the presence of water) into glucose, benzaldehyde and hydro-cyanic acid. The last two substances are both poisons in their own right, but together they work synergistically, i.e. they are more powerful in combination than they are separately. The enzyme that unwraps this package is beta-glucoronidase. This enzyme appears in great quantities in and around cancer cells – but not normal cells. The German doctor Hans Nieper argues that a synthetic version of laetrile, mandelonitrile, might be even more effective.

Laetrile apparently works best on slow growing cancers in the early stages of malignancy. Late stage malignancies need to be slowed down. One way of achieving this is through copper replacement therapy – copper is a vital mineral that is eliminated by cancer cells. Copper supplements help to slow down the respiration rate of the cancer cell and this improves the chances of laetrile working.

Salvestrol

Salvestrols are phytonutrients found in fruits and vegetables – and more so in organic produce – which have only recently been isolated and studied. The results are exciting for people with cancer. The way it works is as follows. Cancer cells contain an enzyme protein called CYP1B1. Professor Burke, the co-discoverer of these phytonutrients, likens this protein to a Trojan horse. If we can find a way of triggering this protein it will release chemicals within the cell that will quickly kill it (the cell). And this is what salvestrols do. They activate this enzyme. Unfortunately, the amount of salvestrols in food is generally insufficient, but a concentrated extract, called Salvestrol, has been developed. It is cheap and widely available on the internet. It is so cheap that it has been proposed that people of all ages should take it simply as a cancer preventative.

Zeolite (Clinoptilolite)

Zeolites are naturally existing, negatively charged minerals, formed by the fusion of glass-rich volcanic rock with either fresh water or sea water. They have a number of rare properties. Clinoptilolite, the zeolite that we are concerned with, has the demonstrated ability to capture and eliminate free radicals, heavy metals, carcinogenic chemicals such as nitrosamines and even viral particles.

So far so good and if this was all that claimed for zeolite, it would be worth taking for these properties alone. And anyone taking it should know that it is generally recognized as having no ill effects whatsoever as long as it does not amount to more than 2% of total food intake. The only caution is that anyone taking it should make sure they are fully hydrated at all times.

However, the big buzz surrounding zeolite is not its detoxification ability but its anti-cancer effects. In animal studies conducted by Dr Ljiljana Bedric, Ph.D., at the Faculty of Veterinary Medicine in Zagreb, Croatia, 51 dogs with various cancers were treated with zeolite. All the dogs improved, some having a dramatic reduction or elimination of their tumours. In only one week, six dogs with prostate cancer were found to be completely tumour free. In human studies 114 patients were given 10–20 grams or more of Megamin capsules containing a specially processed form of zeolite.

The terminal brain cancer patients showed some improvement in their condition within 3 to 4 weeks. Almost all of the 40 lung cancer patients experienced decreased pain and improved respiration within the same time frame. Another 53 patients with terminal gastrointestinal cancers improved but at a much slower rate.

Another group of 16 cancer patients were treated by doctors at the Svecnjak Polyclinic with only Megamin therapy for a period of three years. At the end of the three years, 13 (81%) of the patients were in complete remission. This patient group included three liver cancers, four metastatic melanomas, two bronchial carcinomas, one bladder cancer, and one hepatocellular carcinoma. The other three patients had obtained partial remission and stabilization of their cancers (two lung cancers and one breast cancer).

Megamin can be obtained from *www.megamin.net*. Zeolite is also available in liquid form from the multi-level marketing company Waiora with their product Natural Cell Defence. Destroxin, a powdered form which has the further advantage of being much cheaper, is available from *www.cutcat.com*. Another zeolite product called Denali Green is currently getting a lot of word-of-mouth support. There are testimonials relating to its ability to kill tumours over time. One indication of its power is the fact that many testimonials refer to a Herxheimer response (i.e. the onset of negative symptoms as the first sign of healing). As always, when this happens, cut back the dose or stop taking the product for a few days until the symptoms go.

Pattie McDonald

In May 2002, Pattie, then 58, was diagnosed with breast cancer 'the size of a quarter'. She believes now that contributing factors included being on HRT (Premarin) for six years, long term antibiotic use and a very poor diet ('I was a fast food freak') coupled with a negative outlook on life. Her doctors recommended surgery and radiation.

However, Pattie had a close and trusted friend who had survived ovarian cancer by using bloodroot. She used both bloodroot paste and tonic. The effects of bloodroot quickly revealed that the cancer had already spread to the neck and three lymph nodes.

The Cansema bloodroot paste was applied to the biopsy site on her breast. It took ten days to expel the tumour from her body. As the neck tumours also began to be expelled, Pattie took the tonic and applied paste against the neck. The whole process of treatment took about a month. She experienced excruciating pain and two days of no sleep. (She found out later you should take painkillers.)

In August 2002 she had an MRI that confirmed she was cancer free, and she has remained cancer free four years later. Pattie can be contacted at *pjmacblondie@yahoo.com*.

Attack the Causes of Cancer

The idea that cancer may have a viral cause has been around for many decades. And in fact viruses are now known to be implicated in a great many cancers. Cervical cancer, for example, has been linked to the human papilloma virus (HPV) and is more likely to affect women who have had multiple sex partners. It can also affect virginal nuns, however, so we cannot hypothesize backwards that just because a woman has cervical cancer it must mean that she has had an interesting and varied sex life. But viruses are passed from one person to another and, as always, women are far more vulnerable than men to the viral transactions that take place in the bedroom.

The accusing finger doesn't just stop at viruses. Other theories in the current marketplace of ideas are that cancers are also caused by fungal infections and even parasites.

Let's begin our discussion with fungi. A number of doctors have noted that in the case of leukaemia, the co-presence of a severe fungal infection is extremely common. Intriguingly, treatment with an antifungal drug has also been associated with a number of remissions from cancer. Patrick Quillin, in his book *Beating Cancer with Nutrition*, quotes the story of a well-known oil magnate, 'Doc' Pennington, who was diagnosed with advanced colon cancer in 1972. He got his doctor to prescribe griseofulvin, an antifungal drug, and three months later his cancer had disappeared. He went on to live another 22 years, dying aged 92 in 1994. He founded the Pennington Biomedical Center to study the link between yeast, nutrition and cancer. Research that he funded has shown griseofulvin causes cell death in cancer cells in test tubes.

Dr Tullio Simoncini also believes that cancer is caused by fungus (specifically *Candida albicans*) and treats his patients with 5% solution of sodium bicarbonate injected close to the site of the tumour. For more detailed discussion of his treatment go to *www.curenaturalicancro.com*. He claims this approach is very successful.

The idea that cancer is either caused by fungal infections or actually is a fungal infection is gaining a great deal of strength in some quarters. A number of doctors are reporting that leukaemias, bone cancers and other types of cancer have responded to antifungal cocktails of drugs, and patients have returned when treatment with these drugs has been discontinued too soon. The problem for you, the cancer patient, is to convince your doctor to give you the antifungal drugs.

From fungal infections we turn to viral and bacterial infections. The body's normal response to inflammation is to flood the area with stem calls and various growth factors to aid healing. Where the inflammation, for whatever reason, persists (perhaps because of an irritant or because of low immune function) then these growth factors can transform the stem cells into malignant cells. The teeth, for example, have long been seen as a potential source of such problems, and some doctors in the past have recommended removal of infected teeth for this reason. The other side of the coin is that anti-inflammatory drugs and herbs will tend to be useful in the fight against cancer. Note, however, that pregnancy and cancer are closely related in metabolic terms and anything that works against cancer in this way is likely to lead to the miscarriage of a foetus.

Colloidal silver

One way to attack these viral and bacterial infections is to use colloidal silver. Colloidal silver is a powerful antiseptic and preventative against almost any kind of infection. It disables the enzyme that one-celled bacteria, viruses and fungi need for their oxygen metabolism while in no way harming normal cells. The word 'colloidal' refers to the very fine suspension of silver particles in a solution. Silver is also available in ionic form.

It is also possible that colloidal and/or ionic silver might have a beneficial effect on cancerous tissues, forcing the cancer cells to return to their undifferentiated state. An orthopaedic surgeon, Robert O. Becker, found that a low current (high currents promote cancer growth) passed between two pure silver electrodes – so creating a stream of silver ions between the two electrodes – had the 'side effect' in one of his patients of curing his cancer.

Are there any negative side effects? Ionic silver is generally recognized to be wholly non-toxic. However, the intake of silver salts can eventually lead to a largely cosmetic condition called argyria, in which the skin becomes silvery grey in colour. It must be stressed that there is absolutely no evidence that the intake of pure colloidal or ionic silver will result in argyria. This is a problem only associated with a large intake of silver salts, which can also have a negative neurological impact.

Many people make their own colloidal silver using simple and fairly inexpensive equipment that can be bought on the internet. However, machines that use thin strips of silver wire should be avoided – thick silver rods are best. Store-bought colloidal silver solution can be very variable in quality. It may be better to buy a colloidal silver concentrate and dilute it with distilled water. In this way you have control over the concentration required. For more information about colloidal silver makers go to the Transformation Technologies at *www.braintuner.com.*

The Hulda Clark cure

Hulda Clark has become a famous thorn in the flesh of the American cancer establishment. Her basic thesis has been much derided. It is her view that cancer is caused by a parasite – the human intestinal fluke. This causes no major problems in the gut where it normally resides. But by some means as yet unknown, though associated with the presence of propyl alcohol, it can move to other organs where it starts creating problems. The problem it creates if it gets to the liver is cancer. Her test for cancer is to test for the presence of the marker ortho-phospho-tyrosine (OPT).

All cancer patients, she claims, have both propyl alcohol and the intestinal fluke in their livers. The solvent propyl alcohol is responsible for letting the fluke establish itself in the liver. In order to get cancer, you must have both the parasite and propyl alcohol in your body.

Just as the cause is simple, so is the cure that she proposes: black walnut tincture, wormwood and cloves. The first two kill adult and developmental stages of over 100 parasites. The cloves kill the eggs. They are to be taken as follows:

Black walnut tincture

This should be taken in a glass of water four times a day. Start the first day with one drop each time and increase the dose by one drop a day until on day 20 you are taking 20 drops in water four times a day. Then reduce to 20 drops once a day for 3 months – and then reduce to 30 drops once a day two days a week. It should be taken on an empty stomach, i.e. half an hour before a meal.

Wormwood

This herb is made from the leaves of the artemisia plant. It is also available from herbalists as part of a combination of herbs. It should be taken once a day before the evening meal, increasing daily from one capsule to 14. A lifetime maintenance dose is to take 14 capsules two days a week. Studies have shown that wormwood on its own has demonstrable anti-tumour effects.

Cloves

Obtain whole cloves and grind them up. Cloves that have already been ground do not work. Fill capsules (preferably, size 00 but any vitamin capsules will do) with the ground cloves and take three times a day before meals, building up from one capsule a time to three. Continue until day 10 and then reduce to three capsules once a day for three months – and then just twice a week forever.

Dr Hulda published details of her cure with 100 case studies in her book: *The Cure for all Cancers*. She believes that many, if not most, ailments – from asthma and AIDS to heart disease and schizophrenia – are the result of parasitical infection, and the formula she gives above is one that she believes will rid the body of many of these. She accepts that other formulas will also work. But, in her view, the parasite is only half the problem; the other half is the propyl alcohol. Most people can process this effectively and so it causes no problem whatsoever. But people developing cancer have an impaired ability to do this. She blames the presence in the liver of aflatoxin B. This is a known carcinogenic substance found in mouldy food.

One way to deal with the problem, she argues, is to eliminate propyl alcohol from the system. Unfortunately it is a common ingredient used in the food and cosmetics industries. Check the items in your bathroom and you will find most contain one of the following ingredients: propanol, isopropyl alcohol, isopropanol, and so on. Even if not listed, she claims that propyl alcohol is so commonly used for cleaning industrial equipment that it will very likely be present in minute quantities in a wide range of modern retail goods. But for those people with an impaired ability to break it down, even these quantities are sufficient to cause cancer. She particularly fingers hair and cosmetics products, sugar, carbonated soft drinks and even bottled water, fruit drinks and vitamin supplements. She makes an exception for vitamin C as this helps the liver to break down propyl alcohol by directly attacking the aflatoxin.

Her four-point plan for regaining health is simple but extreme: remove every unnatural chemical substance from your mouth, from your diet, from your body and from your home. She also recommends a zapping device for killing parasites.

Rife machine

Hulda Clark's idea of killing parasites with an electric zapper is not original. Among the earliest pioneers seeking to develop an electronic weapon in the fight against cancer was Royal Raymond Rife (1888–1971), an American inventor. Among his earliest inventions was a microscope through which it was possible to observe living matter (for most microscopes you have to kill what you want to look at and stain it so that salient features become more apparent). From his observations he came to the conclusion that diseases were caused by microbes which could change size, appearing to be a virus one minute and a bacterium the next. He also discovered that these microbes were very vulnerable to energy inputs. He developed the theory that each microbe at each stage in its life cycle had a unique vibrational signature. If you input energy at the same wavelength this would cause the original vibrations to oscillate in an exaggerated way and the result was that the microbe would eventually explode.

He built a machine that could provide energy inputs along a wide range of wavelengths. His machine was tested at the University of Southern California in the early 1930s. Rife reported the results: '16 cases were treated at the clinic for many types of malignancy. After three months, 14 of these so-called hopeless cases were signed off as clinically cured.'

The patients were treated every three days – this was found to be more effective than daily treatment, the reason being that the lymphatic system had to deal with the toxicity created by the dead particles of the virus. In fact all the patients in the study eventually recovered. The machine had a 100% cure rate in cases of terminal cancer.

There is no doubt about the authenticity of the research. So what happened? Why are we not using Rife machines in our hospitals today? The story is that Morris Fishbein, who was not a doctor but headed the American Medical Association and was also a front man for the pharmaceutical industry, was unable to buy into the Rife machine. With the profits of the pharmaceutical industry threatened, he did everything he could to eliminate the machine and was eventually successful.

However some doctors continued to use the machine. In 1940, Dr Arthur Yale reported the results he had obtained using Rife's generator. He reported on four cases that would have been fatal within 90 days. One was a 53-year-old man with a grapefruit-sized tumour in the rectum. Within a week, the pain had gone and within 60 days the entire tumour had disappeared.

A number of machines purporting to be Rife generators are on the market. You can also buy software that claims to convert your own computer into a Rife generator. One issue with these machines is whether analogue is better than digital (almost certainly yes – because with digital outputs there is always a gap between one frequency and the next and microbes will be under evolutionary pressure to occupy these gaps. With analogue machines there are no such gaps).

Another issue that buyers need to consider is whether to have a machine that goes through a pre-set programme of frequencies or whether to take a machine that is programmable to specific frequencies specified for the particular disease.

It seems at first sight that a programmable machine capable of targeting specific disease would be best. Most of these machines will come with a protocol of which frequencies should be used for which health condition. The problem is that there is no general agreement as to which frequencies are specific to cancer. Also, of course, the pressures of evolution will mean that microbes will eventually change frequencies. One researcher, Gary Wade, has solved this problem by creating a machine that has a 45-minute programme that covers all ultrasound frequencies within the relevant range. Whether or not it is curative of cancer is not a subject he is willing to make any comment about.

People undergoing therapy with this machine must make sure they drink plenty of water before and after using the machine. They should also expect to feel tired afterwards. (For more information also see: *www.rifetechnology.com*.)

Stabilized oxygen and sodium chlorite

Serendipity is the word we use when we meet something entirely unexpectedly. You will remember that increasing oxygen to tissues is one way of impeding or even reversing cancer. One product that claims to deliver oxygen to the body is stabilized oxygen, which is in fact a very dilute solution of sodium chlorite (not sodium chloride, which is table salt). Now it is contentious whether or not this product actually does deliver oxygen in a way that is usable by the body. However, that does not mean that stabilized oxygen is potentially useless. In fact it could, if utilized in the correct way, be one of the most powerful anti-cancer weapons in our arsenal.

What happens is that when you mix a few drops of sodium chlorite with vinegar or lemon juice it releases chlorine dioxide. And according to a 1999 statement by the American Society of Analytical Chemists, chlorine dioxide is the most powerful pathogen killer known to man!

Jim Humble, a mining engineer, discovered the powerful healing effects of stabilized oxygen while working in Guyana. He has since developed a more concentrated solution, which he calls Miracle Mineral Supplement. (His story can be found at *www.miraclemineral.org*.) This substance is not only fast acting against malarial parasites and viruses, it also appears (in some cases) at least, to help eliminate cancer. Its mode of action is not clearly understood. It may be that it attacks a viral or fungal cause of cancer or it may be that it reacts explosively in contact with cancerous cells, while remaining completely safe to normal cells. Whatever the case, it is certainly worth giving it a try. Humble recommends starting with a few drops and then slowly increasing by one drop a day until there is a feeling of nausea. This dose level should then be maintained until the nausea (a Herxheimer reaction caused by the body being temporarily overcome by toxins released by the healing or curative process) is no longer felt. It is then possible to continue increasing the dose. (Miracle Mineral Supplement is inexpensive and available from *www.globallight.net.*)

Elonna McKibben

In 1989, having taken fertility treatment, Elonna found herself pregnant with quintuplets. However, as the pregnancy progressed, Elonna began feeling deep-seated pains. It was eventually discovered, after the birth of her children, that the pains were not a side effect of her pregnancy – the exceptional nature of which had camouflaged the fact that she had a tumour in her spinal cord.

This was diagnosed as stage 4 glioblastoma multiforme (GBM), a very rare and invariably fatal cancer. 'As mine was in the spinal cord,' Elonna wrote later, 'it made it even more rare, more aggressive and faster killing. I was told I would not survive long enough to see my children's first birthday.'

If that was not bad enough, the combined effect of the surgery and cancer had left her paralysed from the waist down. When their bone marrow chemotherapy suggestion was refused, her doctors recommended radiation but stated that, at best, it would only slightly delay the inevitable.

Fortunately, someone who read about her situation from the

news coverage her family was receiving contacted her husband, Rob, and sent him a video about CanCell (also known as Protocell). Elonna was naturally very sceptical: 'If there was a cure for cancer, don't you think they would be using it instead of letting thousands of people die.'

However, she started taking it on the basis that she had nothing to lose and everything to gain. Its effects were quickly obvious. 'I began to eliminate the cancer waste product about 18 hours after my first dose. It literally poured out of me: I threw it up; my bowel movements were extremely loose, stringy and frequent throughout the day; I lost it in my urine; my nose ran so much I had to keep a tissue with me at all times; I sweated it out profusely; I had hot/cold flushes and night sweats. When the nurses would give me a sponge bath after a night sweat, the water would be a golden brown colour with what they referred to as "tapioca balls" floating in it.'

Believing these effects to be a clear sign that CanCell was working, she persevered with it. After several weeks she found she was feeling much better. Christmas came and went and she started to do physical therapy to help her mobility. Then in February 1990 she went and had scans to see what was happening. The radiologist was stunned to find no trace of the cancer. Although cancer-free, Elonna continued the CanCell treatment for a further two years.

As of March 2008, Elonna McKibben is still alive and her full story can be read on her website at *www.elonnamckibben.com*.

Open Yourself to Possibilities

We are now approaching the end of this brief journey. I hope that, along the way, you have come to see that what is amazing is not that alternative approaches can cure cancer, but that there are so many alternative cancer approaches that appear to promise so much and have either scientific support or the anecdotal testimony of individuals. The question is: why are these approaches not offered by our cancer clinics? Why must so many people suffer and die, and do so in ignorance of the possibilities around them? Sadly, until there is a large groundswell of public opinion, there will be no improvement in the situation. But more and more people are becoming aware that the alternative approaches do have credibility and are worth exploring – and doctors are having to respond to this movement. Change is inevitable and it will come.

But, to return to the present, if you have cancer and you have read the previous chapters you will be facing the dilemma of which therapies to follow. I must remind you of a point that I made at the start of this book. Many, if not all, of these therapies are effective. In that they are effective, they can have a strong impact on the body. The first stage of that impact will be the appearance of negative symptoms as the cancer tumour begins to disintegrate. It is not good for the body to have to deal with too much toxicity too quickly – especially as it is in a weakened state already. Therefore build up your own anti-cancer strategy slowly. Don't attack with too many weapons all at once. Be a little bit patient. Choose the therapies that you instinctively respond to.

And it may be that you will need some help. I believe that anyone who is seriously ill with a chronic condition such as cancer will benefit from having the personal support of others. There may be cancer support groups in your area, but in my view these need to be approached cautiously. Just because there is a cancer support group doesn't mean that it will be useful to join.

What is it that you should look for in a cancer group? Well, first of all you must try to establish if there is any underlying agenda – is it run by a local hospital, for example? If so, then it may be resistant to ideas about alternative approaches.

However, you don't have to go out to look for pre-existing cancer support groups in the community, you can create your own. I would like to suggest that your own cancer support group should consist of two or three friends (not too many, even one will do) who will be there not because they have cancer but because they want to help you. You should ask them to read this book too – give them their own copies – and work through the various strategies, discussing them. Let your friends do some of the reading that you may not feel up to. Invite your friends to breakfast every Saturday morning (or whenever is more convenient) for a sharing session – a session for sharing not just what is in your mind but also what is in your heart.

There are support groups on the web as well. I certainly recommend the Yahoo health groups. The Cancercured and Flaxoil2 groups are both very active.

Many of the references in this book are to internet websites. Also, many of the supplements recommended in these pages are easily obtained from internet suppliers. If you are not personally computer literate this may pose a problem. When choosing your support group think of who might be able to help directly or indirectly in accessing these websites and suppliers – by themselves being computer literate or by knowing someone who is.

I leave you with that thought and with some suggestions for follow-up reading.

First of all I would recommend that you read my more complete work, *Cancer: The Complete Recovery Guide*, which goes into a great deal more detail on all the subjects that I have touched on in this book and much more. For information as to its availability go to *www.fightingcancer.com*.

If, despite everything you have read here, you wish to get further details of what the most up-to-date orthodox treatments are for your cancer, then go to the following American National Cancer Institute website and look for the pdq files at *www.cancer.gov/cancertopics*.

Lastly, it remains for me to wish you success in your own personal fight with cancer.

Further Reading

For those who would like some background on the medical context I would like to recommend the following books:

Ralph Moss, *The Cancer Industry*, Equinox Press, New York 1996 (This book is a must!)

Robert Procter, *Cancer Wars: How Politics shapes what we know and don't know about cancer*, Basic Books, New York 1995

Dean Black, *Health at the Crossroads*, Tapestry Press, Utah 1988

And for personal testimony:

Norman Cousins, *An Anatomy of An Illness as Perceived by the Patient*, W.W. Norton & Co, New York 1979

Beata Bishop, *My Triumph Over Cancer*, Keats Publishing 1985

Michael Gearin-Tosh, *Living Proof, A Medical Mutiny*, Simon & Schuster, London 2002

Anne Frahm, *The Cancer Battle Plan*, Pinon Press, Colorado 1993

Caryl Hirshberg and Marc Barasch, *Remarkable Recovery*, Headline, London 1995

There are many other books worth reading, but these will provide as good a platform as any for your new life-long interest in cancer.

Other books mentioned in the text:

Angell, Marcia, *The Truth About the Drug Companies – How they deceive us and what to do about it*, Random House, New York 2004

Bakan, Joel, *The Corporation*, Constable & Robinson, London 2004

Becker, Robert, *Cross Currents*, Jeremy P. Tarcher, New York 1991

Chamberlain, Jonathan, *Fighting Cancer: A Survival Guide*, Hodder Headline, London 1996

Chamberlain, Jonathan, *Cancer: The Complete Recovery Guide*, e-book, 2007 *www.fightingcancer.com*

Chopra, Deepak, *Quantum Healing*, Bantam Books, New York 1989

Clark, Hulda, *The Cure for All Cancers*, ProMotion Publishing, California 1993

Corbin-Wheeler, Felicity, *God's Healing Word*, Book Publishing World, 2006

Gawler, Ian, *You Can Conquer Cancer*, Michelle Anderson Publishing, 2001

Kassirer, Jerome, *On The Take – How medicine's complicity with big business can endanger your health*, Oxford University Press, New York 2005

Quillin, Patrick, *Beating Cancer with Nutrition*, Nutrition Times Press Inc., 2005

Schulze, Richard, *There Are No Incurable Diseases*, Natural Healing Publications, 1999

Weston, Percy, *Cancer: Cause and Cure*, Bookbin Publishing, Adelaide 2000

Index